THE MEDICAL & SURGICAL

Residency Survival Guide

T0178787

How to Build a Tactical Advantage for Success

Daniel McMahon

The Medical & Surgical Residency Survival Guide: *How to Build a Tactical Advantage for Success*

tfm Publishing Limited, Castle Hill Barns, Harley, Shrewsbury, SY5 6LX, UK
Tel: +44 (0)1952 510061; Fax: +44 (0)1952 510192
E-mail: info@tfmpublishing.com; Web site: www.tfmpublishing.com

Editing, design & typesetting: Nikki Bramhill BSc Hons Dip Law
Cover photos: © iStock.com
First class medical team (PeopleImages) — Stock photo ID:869288118

First edition:	© 2019
Paperback	ISBN: 978-1-910079-67-6
E-book editions:	2019
ePub	ISBN: 978-1-910079-68-3
Mobi	ISBN: 978-1-910079-69-0
Web pdf	ISBN: 978-1-910079-70-6

Printed by Gutenberg Press Ltd., Gudja Road, Tarxien, GXQ 2902, Malta
Tel: +356 2398 2201; Fax: +356 2398 2290
E-mail: info@gutenberg.com.mt; Web site: www.gutenberg.com.mt

Contents

page

FOREWORD   vii

ABOUT THE AUTHOR   xi

SPECIAL THANKS   xiii

DEDICATION   xv

REVIEWS   xvi

PART I RULES OF ENGAGEMENT —
CALIBRATE YOUR BRAIN FOR SUCCESS

Chapter 1   It's a grind — play the long game   3

Chapter 2   Perseverance & endurance   11

Chapter 3   Mental strength & fortitude   19

Chapter 4   Availability, affability, & ability   27

Chapter 5   There is no substitute for experience   33

PART II HOW TO PLAY THE GAME

Chapter 6   Triage & preparation   45

Chapter 7   Delegate   53

Chapter 8   Use the chain of command   57

Chapter 9   Ask for help   63

Chapter 10 Avoid drama like the plague   69

Chapter 11 Don't forget the administrative minutiae   75

PART III PROFESSIONALISM

Chapter 12 Professional appearance & behavior   83

Chapter 13 Communication   89

Chapter 14 Integrity & character   97

Chapter 15 Check your ego at the door   103

Chapter 16 Arrogance, braggadocious, &   107

             the surgical dragon

Chapter 17 Roundsmanship   115

Chapter 18 The morbidity & mortality conference   119

PART IV TALKING TO PATIENTS & FAMILIES

Chapter 19 Lay it out in layman's terms   141

Chapter 20 Delivering bad news   147

Chapter 21 Empathy   153

PART V PROVIDER WELLNESS

Chapter 22 Nutrition   161

Chapter 23 Exercise   165

Chapter 24 Sleep   169

Chapter 25 Work hard, play hard, & better living   173
           through chemistry?

Chapter 26 Physician burnout   181

PART VI FAMILY, FRIENDS, & FINANCES

Chapter 27 Family & friends   189

Chapter 28 Finances   195

PART VII ONGOING EDUCATION

Chapter 29 Read one hour per day   203

Chapter 30 Research   209

Chapter 31 Professional organizations & societies   213

PART VIII MENTOR, TEACH, & LEAD

Chapter 32 Mentorship   217

Chapter 33 Teach   223

Chapter 34 Lead   227

AFTERWORD   233

Foreword

As a prior surgical resident, and now as a junior surgical attending, I felt compelled to write about the unique challenges, trials, and tribulations of medical residency and surgical training while the faint bruising from my training remained and had not yet completely faded. One never forgets an experience of this magnitude; however, I wanted to translate my thoughts on the matter into print while they actively lingered among the neurons of my cerebral cortex.

As I launched into this project it was my intent to write a book, not as a braggadocious memoir about the "great cases" I experienced during my training, nor my personal accolades, but rather a focused, honest, and straightforward text regarding the unique challenges encountered in residency training and how one may employ a number of strategies to facilitate tactful navigation of these challenging waters.

One of my primary goals as I approached writing this book was to draft an easily digestible and relatively abbreviated volume that drives the important points home without a bunch of worthless fodder. The formative years of your training certainly bring an enormous amount of challenging reading and I believe you will find the following text easily navigable and high yield. I personally find that the books or readings that have the greatest influence upon my life and psyche are short and sweet and have the ability to be revisited on a regular basis with value added after each subsequent reading. I humbly hope to have instilled these same characteristics with this offering.

Certainly, some of the tenets and principles discussed apply to life in general; however, I would like to offer my personal insight and opinions on how these topics specifically apply to you as a medical resident or surgical trainee. Depending on your particular field of training, some of these chapters may be more applicable to your chosen pursuit of study than others. That being said, whether you are training in a surgical specialty, obstetrics and gynecology, primary care, anesthesiology, emergency medicine, pediatrics, radiology, or even pathology, I believe each of the following chapters will contain some degree of useful insight for you to draw from despite the vast differences among the numerous disciplines of medicine and surgery.

Medical residency and surgical training are without a doubt enormously challenging endeavors, rife with sacrifices that must be endured for the individual progressing through the training as well as family members and friends of the individual muscling through the training, day after day, month after month, and year after year. While medical residency is one of the most unique and rigorous mentally and physically demanding training pipelines known in the professional world, the rewards are certainly worth the toil.

The vast amount of information you must assimilate and digest, as well as the technical skills you must command mastery of in medical residency and surgical training, are analogous to drinking from a fire hose. This training is a gauntlet of professional development that must be courageously navigated with patience, perseverance, endurance, discipline, grit, tenacity, integrity, professionalism, boundless energy, empathy, and an intrepid drive that at times must be summoned from the darkest reaches of your soul to continue moving forward.

By this point in your training you have succeeded in college and medical school. Maybe you are already progressing through a challenging residency program or maybe you have found yourself embarking upon a challenging fellowship. Regardless, I hope the thoughts expressed in the following text will spur some degree of self-reflection and enable you to construct a mental armamentarium of weaponry that will facilitate successful navigation through your seemingly endless training pipeline.

You may find some of this advice frank, blunt, and brutally honest. Well, so is real life and so is medicine when you are dealing with real patients who are sick, terribly injured, or dying. Medicine and surgery are a full-contact sport. Grow a thick skin, put on your armor, and head to the fight.

I hope that as you read through these pages you will absorb a few words of advice from someone who has experienced exactly what you are going through or what you may be preparing yourself to go through. I openly admit to making more mistakes than I wish to count throughout the course of my training. Fortunately, this project has forced me to cathartically reflect upon many of those mistakes.

It is my sincere wish that at least a few of these short chapters will come to your aid in maintaining an even keel throughout your training and prevent you from making some of the same painful mistakes I naively committed.

Are you up for it? Are you ready to take the helm and chart a course through the challenges of your training that are inevitably waiting in the shadows and nebulously shimmering on the horizon? Absolutely! There is no time like the present. Let's get moving.

About the author

Daniel McMahon is a native of Fairhope, Alabama. He received an undergraduate degree in biology from the University of Alabama and was awarded a Navy Health Professions Scholarship to complete his Doctor of Medicine training at the University of Alabama School of Medicine.

Following medical school he completed general surgery internship training at the Naval Medical Center Portsmouth, Virginia, prior to a course of aerospace medical and flight training at the Naval Aerospace Medical Institute in Pensacola, Florida, where he was designated a naval flight surgeon.

After flight surgery training he completed a two-year operational flight surgery tour while based in Lemoore, California, with Carrier Air Wing Eleven. During this tour, he embarked aboard the aircraft carrier, USS Nimitz, in support of carrier strike group exercises and fleet operations. He was also deployed with Carrier Air Wing Fourteen, aboard USS Ronald

Reagan, in support of Operation Enduring Freedom and Operation Iraqi Freedom.

Following his flight surgery tour, he went on to complete general surgery residency training at the Naval Medical Center Portsmouth, Virginia. At the conclusion of his formal surgical training he completed a two-year overseas tour as a staff general surgeon at the Naval Hospital Yokosuka, Japan, where he served as the Department Head for the Department of General Surgery. Additionally, during this overseas tour he was deployed as Officer-in-Charge of an austere expeditionary surgical team in support of Naval Special Operations forces.

Shortly after this overseas tour of duty he was deployed to Afghanistan to serve as a forward trauma surgeon in support of ongoing coalition operations.

He is a member of the American College of Surgeons as well as the Excelsior Surgical Society and is an Assistant Professor of Surgery with the Uniformed Services University of Health Sciences.

He currently lives in Mobile, Alabama, with his wife Aurelia and his two children, Benton and Aurelia Marie, where he enjoys hunting, fishing, and spending time with friends and family.

Special thanks

A special thanks to Nikki Bramhill of TFM Publishing for enthusiastically taking this project on board without hesitation and with open arms. Thanks to her dedication the publishing process for this project has truly been a wonderful and enjoyable experience for an initially apprehensive first-time author. Her professionalism and attention to detail are clearly evident in the finished project. I owe Nikki a great debt of gratitude for all her hard work that could never be effectively repaid nor reciprocated.

I also want to thank Martin Hill, of MPHC Marketing, for believing in the idea of this book and putting his expertise to work into the marketing campaign for this project.

I would like to thank all of the teachers, mentors, military leaders, and medical educators who have had such an important and profound impact upon my life. You have helped me to become the surgeon and military officer I am today.

A heartfelt thank you to all of my family, friends, and colleagues who have been so very generous and have brought so much richness to my personal and professional lives.

Dedication

This book is dedicated to my mother, father, wife, and children:

To my sweet, dear mother. You have always been a devoted educator and a compassionate volunteer. You have taught your boys the enduring joy and happiness that can be gained from upholding and living the virtues of kindness, politeness, and altruism.

To my father. You have selflessly and tirelessly worked so very hard to provide a wonderful and happy life for your family. Leading by example, you have taught your sons the utmost importance of a strong work ethic and the everlasting merits of integrity by directly displaying these invaluable character traits in your own actions.

To my wonderful and beautiful wife. You have faithfully stood by my side and have been a source of perpetual strength and support through the tumultuous peaks and valleys of surgical training and military service.

To my adorable children. You are too young to realize this now, but I hope one day you will truly know how much happiness, joy, and warmth you bring to my life.

Reviews

Dr. McMahon has meaningfully articulated the overarching and salient principles of engagement for successful training in medical and surgical residency. The sage advice and directives provided by the highly regarded author and educator provides emerging perspectives that advantage the young physician entering a specialty that offers considerable variability in its educational content. It is highly recommended for its comprehensive focus that embodies the principles for resident and student success to maximize advantages in residency training and subsequent practice for the art and science of medicine or surgery.

"The Medical & Surgical Residency Survival Guide: How to Build a Tactical Advantage for Success" embodies the authoritative compass to direct all levels of obligation and expectations for the professional student/resident following their acceptance of the highest level of responsibility expectant of humanity — a physician — who by definition has assumed the most arduous and responsibility-laden task that can befall an individual. The author has been most successful in formulating, within eight sections, the 34 chapters that provide foundational advice for medical students and medical/surgical residents with their directives and expectations of the different levels of commitment, responsibility, and accountability. Encouraged as a "must-read" text for one considering entry to medical school and as the requisite text for the student entering accredited residency training. **Kirby I. Bland MD FACS, Professor of Surgery and Chair Emeritus, UAB Department of Surgery, Birmingham Alabama, USA.**

Residency can be a time of wonder, learning and fulfilment; or, alternatively, anxiety, stress, and panic. Like everything in life, learning some easy rules to follow, and some little tricks, can make your life more like the former, and less like the latter. Why would you not read this book before approaching your residency? **Jonothan J. Earnshaw DM FRCS, Editor in Chief, *British Journal of Surgery*.**

ALL medical trainees repeatedly face complex decisions and challenges in the educational environment. This novel little book is chock-full of survival advice and practical points for interacting with the many professors, peers, colleagues, critics, and observers of the almost continuous rites of passage. It is best read in short excerpts, just before a targeted encounter to maximally learn lessons recorded by others in similar conditions. Many of the tidbits of advice are similar and often repeated, as the "survival pearls" are often very similar and worthy of being remembered. **Kenneth L. Mattox MD, Distinguished Service Professor, Michael E. DeBakey Department of Surgery, Baylor College of Medicine, and Chief of Staff/Chief of Surgery at the Ben Taub General Hospital, Houston, Texas, USA.**

Dr. McMahon's book, "The Medical & Surgical Residency Survival Guide" provides a compact and easy-to-read guide to succeeding during residency, with practical and honest advice on how to balance the rigors of medical/surgical training and personal care needs. No matter your specialty, you will benefit from heeding the advice contained in this book, which would maximize both the educational opportunities during training, as well as your overall professional development. I wish such a book were available when I first started residency myself! As a physician-mentor who works closely with international medical students, I find this book especially useful for international medical graduates who will pursue postgraduate clinical training in the United States. **Kris "Siri" Siriratsivawong MD FACS, General Surgeon, Department of Medical Education, Showa University, Tokyo, Japan.**

Beginning residency training is an intimidating venture in the best of circumstances. While well prepared in the basics of medical care, the actual "how to" do much of anything can be elusive if not downright impossible to discern for the new resident. A good go to handbook that offers a game plan for the long haul with advice about specific hurdles along the way would be a major benefit to the junior and intermediate level resident.

Dr. McMahon, recently graduated from a general surgical residency, provides such a handbook. The text is short and to the point. In his forward Dr. McMahon is clear that his goal is to drive home important points that will allow the resident physician to be successful both professionally and personally. Each chapter addresses a specific aspect of residency training, emphasizes why it is important and suggests strategies for coping with the physical and emotional stresses imposed. The book is divided into parts with labels like "Rules of Engagement" and "Professionalism". Chapters talk about how to talk to patients and their families, an especially difficult task when dealing with advanced diseases or complications. Equally important are chapters that address how to maintain your own sanity. How do you protect your own wellness and that of loved ones and friends around you? How you deal with your finances is an excellent addition to this text as it is often overlooked. The book concludes with thoughts on how to assure your continuing education, something necessary for the rest of your life. Lastly, is the reminder that as physicians we are called on to develop the next generation and to embrace that mentorship task enthusiastically.

This book is a quick read with short chapters that facilitate just in time reading when looking for fast advice. Dr. McMahon's style is concise and shows his military background but is laced with real experiences that drive home the points being made. This book fills a real void and is a worthwhile addition to the reading of any junior or intermediate level resident. The text is at times humorous, at times reminiscent of difficult clinical circumstances, but consistently pointing the way to successful and fulfilling completion of residency training and launching a post residency career. **Leonard J. Weireter Jr. MD FACS, Professor, School of Health Professions, Medical Director of the Sentara Center for Simulation and Immersive Learning, Eastern Virginia Medical School, Norfolk, VA, USA.**

Part I

RULES OF ENGAGEMENT – CALIBRATE YOUR BRAIN FOR SUCCESS

You can never cross the ocean until you have the courage to lose sight of the shore.

Christopher Columbus

Chapter 1

It's a grind — play the long game

Rome wasn't built in a day.

There is no way around it. Medical residency and surgical training is an all-out grind. You will progress through one morning of rounding at a time, one day at a time, one night at a time, and one shift at a time. You will endure one clinic patient, one inpatient or emergency department consult, one trauma alert, one procedure, or one operation at a time. You will press on one week at a time, one month at a time, and one year at a time. You get the idea. This is an ultra-marathon not a sprint.

At times your training will seem like an indefinite apprenticeship that is rife with challenges and unforeseen obstacles along the way. The price required to complete your training is steep and will include blood, sweat, tears, and

At times your training will seem

like an indefinite apprenticeship

that is rife with challenges

and unforeseen obstacles

along the way.

sacrifice. There are also great rewards along the way. Do not forget that. And yes, your training is a means to an end.

"What is the end result," you ask?

The end result is to be a confident, competent, intelligent, capable, successful, and well-rounded physician in whatever field of medicine you strive to become board-certified.

Like medical school, residency is a grind but on an entirely different level. The level of responsibility is vastly different in internship and residency than what most experience in medical school. While you are not the attending physician of the patients you will be caring for, you are directly responsible for the day to day execution of patient care at the ground level. From inpatient to outpatient responsibilities, and everything in between, you will carry the lion's share of direct patient contact among a large cadre of physicians in whatever institution you find yourself training.

You will order medications, laboratory studies, and radiographic studies. You will work among a wide array of different clinical services depending on your path of training. You will perform inpatient rounds, see inpatient consults, and experience a litany of outpatient clinical encounters. You will write thousands of patient notes, consultation reports, discharge summaries, and operative reports. You will chase down lab results, imaging studies, and consultation advice like a bloodhound in hot pursuit of *Cool Hand Luke*. You will perform procedures and operations. You will change dressings and place lines, tubes, and drains. The list goes on and on.

In addition to all of this clinical work, you will prepare for lectures, presentations, academic conferences, and board examinations. You will work in a measure of academic research and maintain some semblance of a personal life outside the grasp of the black hole that will be your training as a medical or surgical house officer. You will work eighty hours a week on average; sometimes more and sometimes less.

Get the idea? You will constitute the backbone of direct patient care throughout your residency training and all the while you will maintain your sanity and drive to tread on.

Take this seriously. Your patients and your medical team are depending on you. You would not have made it to this level, or be performing at this level, if you did not take things seriously. However, we all get tired, complacent, and burned out which at times requires us to remember this is not just a game we are slugging through.

This is real life and these are real people with real illnesses. This is real pathology and these are real traumatic injuries with patients desperately clinging to life. These are real patients who are anesthetized under hot operating room lights and lying on a cold operating table. Their lives are in your hands and there are real consequences awaiting one false move if you do not stay at the top of your game.

You must commit to the long game. Residency is a slow burn. Completing your training does not magically occur overnight.

You must commit to the long game. Residency is a slow burn. Completing your training does not magically occur overnight.

Seek to execute realistic goals in the short term to achieve unrealistic goals in the long term. Sometimes the realistic short-term goal is merely dragging yourself through the wee hours of a thirty-six-hour call shift as a means to bringing the unrealistic long-term goal of completing your residency training to fruition.

You must transform this seemingly insurmountable and monstrous task into many small tasks that you can more easily approach and chisel away at one swing at a time. You cannot eat an eighteen-ounce steak in one bite. It takes many small bites and it takes time. If you try to swallow a whole steak in one bite or engulf your training whole like a hungry macrophage juiced up on cytokines you will choke and asphyxiate. Confront this training process one day, one night, one shift, one patient, one consult, and one operation at a time. You must approach this behemoth in small digestible bites lest it will consume you and your sanity.

Confront this training process

one day, one night, one shift, one

patient, one consult, and one

operation at a time.

Throughout residency you must learn to live in the moment. Be the best you can be in the moment and execute to the best of your ability in that moment with intense laser-like focus. Learn to harness and utilize this focus for every clinical question thrown at you, during every patient encounter, with every history and physical you write, with every incision you make, with every suture you place and tie, and with every electrocardiogram or chest film you read.

> *Be the best you can be in the*
>
> *moment and execute to the best*
>
> *of your ability in that moment*
>
> *with intense laser-like focus.*

You cannot waste time constantly worrying about the end result or you will not react, act accordingly, and execute in the here and now. Do not find yourself continuously ruminating about the end result or what lies ahead. Things will take care of themselves and things will fall into place as long as you tackle what is standing right in front of you, right there in the clear and present, and keep pressing forward.

Conversely, during this lengthy training pipeline you must remind yourself of the big picture by mentally breaking things down on a very simplistic level and seeing things from a thirty-thousand-foot view rather than right up close. Take a step back and zoom out from time to time. Learn how to keep the big picture centered in view as your main focal point, rather than being distracted and confused by every last-minute detail exhaustingly vying for your attention.

If this is interpreted as doom and gloom it is not meant to be. This is meant to be realistic, honest, and authentic. Take the challenges of your training head-on. Take the bull by the horns and you will reap the rewards hand over fist from how gratifying the practice of medicine and surgery can be if you take it one step at a time and be the best you can be with each small step along the way.

Some call us crazy for willingly taking this kind of a commitment on board. Maybe we are a little crazy to endure this training but remember that the sacrifice will be worth the rewards. Your training is a noble and worthy adversary. You will succeed in becoming a soldier against pathology, pain, suffering, illness, and injury. You have a gift and a drive to achieve that most folks cannot even begin to fathom. Go out and show the world what you have got. You will reach the summit and you will become a much stronger person as you progress along the path that will ultimately lead to the culmination of your medical training.

You have a gift and a drive to achieve that most folks cannot even begin to fathom. Go out and show the world what you have got.

Chapter 2

Perseverance & endurance

Aut inveniam viam aut faciam.

~ I shall either find a way

or make one.

I have had the unique and amazing experience of working with, and deploying with, the Naval Special Warfare — Navy SEAL — community during my military service. I learned several invaluable lessons about perseverance and endurance from these elite warriors that I think are well worth taking on board. Take these lessons on board as a medical resident or surgical trainee who is battling it out day by day in the trenches of clinical warfare wielding only a stethoscope and a reflex hammer as your sole weapons of force protection. These lessons will challenge you to approach life on an entirely different level and will change your life for the better if you commit to them. These powerful nuggets of knowledge and motivation are as follows:

First:

Remove "I can't" from your vocabulary. By simply mumbling the words "I can't" you are accepting defeat before you ever take the first steps in executing a goal, task, or mission. Eliminate "I can't" right out of your head space and incinerate it with impunity. Let others say "I can't," and thank them for it because they are opening space for you to take the world head on and exude success from every fiber and pore of your being.

> *Remove "I can't" from*
>
> *your vocabulary.*

You are not a defeatist. You have the guts, the strength, the endurance, the courage, and the perseverance to do what it takes. Saying, "I can't," is really just feeling sorry for yourself because you do not think you are good enough. You have got what it takes. When you purge "I can't" from your vocabulary, you will gain the upper ground and possess a powerful and tactical mental advantage that will allow you to posture, attack, execute, and conquer your training.

Second:

Sustain the mental attitude, "You will have to kill me before I quit." If you have true purpose and are truly committed to doing this and doing this right, you will either do it or die trying. This may sound a little extreme when we are talking about completing medical residency or surgical training as this is not actual military combat. That is quite true. However, committing to this ethos will frame your attitude into one of perseverance and endurance that few can attest to and will ensure your success in completing residency with unrivaled performance and an outstanding attitude.

> *Sustain the mental attitude,*
>
> *"You will have to kill me*
>
> *before I quit."*

Third:

When you think you have hit a wall or that you are at the brink of complete physical exhaustion, you have only exhausted forty percent of your true capacity. If you find yourself halfway through a call night thinking you cannot possibly make it through another minute, one more call from the transfer center, one more page from the ICU or floor, one more consult from the ED, or one more emergent operation, remember the forty-percent rule. Keep digging deep. You have got what it takes. Keep grinding forward. Take a deep breath and push on; one foot in front of the other. Do you want to be an elite warrior or just some schmuck who cannot hack it?

> *When you think you have hit a wall or that you are at the brink of complete physical exhaustion, you have only exhausted forty percent of your true capacity.*

There will be days when you think you might not be able to power through. When this occurs, you must find the motivational spark that is waiting to be lit somewhere deep in that cerebral cortex of yours. Be able to reproduce that mental spark of motivation and be able to access it readily. Is it your spouse, your children, your family, your friends, or your spiritual life? Is it money, fame, or fortune? Whatever it may be, tap into that spark of motivation when you need it most, when you are at the verge of feeling sorry for yourself, and when the thoughts of quitting start to creep in.

Whatever it may be, tap into

that spark of motivation when

you need it most

Tap into that spark of motivation when you are running on fumes and let it power you through the trying times when it sucks and you feel like giving up. These are the times when you have to find your stride and separate yourself from the rest of the pack. When you reach deep and tap into that spark of motivation and inspiration, you can channel this into action and intensity, pivotally regain traction, and march onward to victory.

Do not settle for mediocrity or failure. If you find yourself settling, you assuredly have not put out one-hundred percent of the true effort you possess and as a result you will not achieve the goals you have set for yourself. Dig in your heels, put out, and lay it all on the line. If you do not emerge victorious you will have no one to blame but yourself and you will regret it when the din of battle abates and there are no second chances in sight. Walk away the proud victor instead of the defeated who is hobbling away with his tail between his legs.

Do not settle for mediocrity

or failure.

Never allow yourself to become despondent about the negative vicissitudes of the progression through your medical training which will inevitably occur daily if not multiple times daily; for these trials and tribulations will foster personal growth, perseverance, character, resilience, and success. Without attacking the challenges that arise along the way and must be dealt with head-on and navigated with courage and creativity, one becomes flat, complacent, ungrateful, and weak. Do not become so deeply bogged down in your own sorrow when challenges arise that you cannot dig yourself out, pick yourself up, and keep moving forward.

Do not feel sorry for yourself when the going gets tough. No one else is going to feel sorry for you. So why should you waste time feeling sorry for yourself? If anyone else does carve out time to feel sorry for you it will not last long. They have their own shit to deal with rather than worrying about yours and they will be moving on.

> *Do not feel sorry for yourself*
>
> *when the going gets tough.*

No one is going to make this happen for you. You have to want it. You have to taste it. Go out there, get after it, and chase it down with intensity like your hair is on fire. Do not take no for an answer, take no prisoners, and find a way to get it done.

In the immortal words of Admiral Farragut during the battle of Mobile Bay in the Civil War, "Damn the torpedoes, full speed ahead!"

No one is going to make this

happen for you. You have to

want it. You have to taste it.

Go out there, get after it, and

chase it down with intensity like

your hair is on fire.

Chapter 3

Mental strength & fortitude

Pain is weakness leaving

the body.

There is no question that at times throughout the course of your medical training you will have to rely on brute mental strength and fortitude to win the day. You have to be mentally strong and let the almost constant barrage of small arms fire roll off your back. Larger artillery rounds impacting upon your fox-hole may take a little more work to press through but they will not stop you from executing the mission at hand and being successful.

We have all heard the phrase, "Don't sweat the small stuff." This is no different in medical training as it is in the larger context of life. You do not have time to worry about the "small

There is no question that at times throughout the course of your medical training you will have to rely on brute mental strength and fortitude to win the day.

stuff." You have to keep moving forward in spite of the constant background static created by the "small stuff." The show must go on.

You will be yelled at, scoffed at, and scolded by attendings, fellows, and senior residents as well as nurses, support staff, and even patients from time-to-time. If there is important and constructive feedback flowing from these sometimes stern rebukes, then by all means listen and take that information on

"Don't sweat the small stuff."

board to improve yourself. But if not, screw them, or insert a more colorful word instead of screw if you please.

These folks coming down on you, whoever they are, will move past whatever bunched their underpants into a wad in short order. They will probably forget about whatever it was they were barking or squawking about in a matter of minutes. There is no need for you to worry about or carry that mental garbage around in your head space all day. You have got more important things to take care of, including yourself. When this happens just smile and say, "Copy that." Take any constructive feedback that is warranted on board and move on.

An adage often heard from numerous elite military training communities is, "Pain is weakness leaving the body." As cliché as it sounds we have heard this as a similar cliché our entire lives and it is true: "What doesn't kill you makes you stronger." There is no better fit for these frequently used but no-nonsense and simplistic adages than medical residency and surgical training.

One of our most basic human instincts which rests at the core of human nature is to avoid pain and discomfort. However, taking that pain and discomfort on head-first, and there is plenty to go around in medical training, is the key to unlocking your true success as a house officer. "No pain, no gain." There is one of those corny clichés again, but how true it is.

Put yourself out there and take a calculated leap of faith. It may hurt, it may be difficult, and it may make you feel vulnerable. That is okay. We spend so much time protecting ourselves from things that seem difficult and challenging that we prevent ourselves from progressing mentally, physically, emotionally, or spiritually and we prevent ourselves from maximizing our full potential.

We spend so much time protecting ourselves from things that seem difficult and challenging that we prevent ourselves from progressing mentally, physically, emotionally, or spiritually and we prevent ourselves from maximizing our full potential.

You may be afraid of making a mistake, be afraid of being wrong, or be afraid of being embarrassed in front of your colleagues or your attendings. That is okay. If you have a question about a clinical scenario or do not know the answer to a clinical question, chances are that most of your colleagues standing around will not know either. Be the one who steps out of the door onto the field of combat first. Take the shot at a tough question, ask the question that everyone else is afraid of asking, or take on a difficult task that everyone else is afraid of. By having the courage to simply take the first step forward onto the clinical battlefield you can capitalize on that momentum, conquer the objective that stands before you, and win the day.

Take the shot at a tough question, ask the question that everyone else is afraid of asking, or take on a difficult task that everyone else is afraid of.

These things that intimidate us, these things that we hide from, these things that seem scary or seem painful, typically do not end up being nearly as awful as we dreamt them up to be in our own scheming little minds anyway. Now, there is a distinct difference between putting yourself out there and taking calculated risks versus being completely reckless. Please do not confuse these two entirely different things.

To employ mental toughness and fortitude you must find the primal instinct and visceral drive in your core to attack whatever may be forcing you to retreat from the line to establish a defensive rather than an offensive front. Once you accost and directly confront an obstacle in your path of training you can decisively turn the tables and take the offensive approach rather than cowering in a defensive posture. Once you assume the offensive tack you then possess positive control of the situation.

Attack and diffuse these obstacles that will be hiding along your path in medical training rather than allowing them to suppress your forward momentum. Do not be afraid of them. As you willingly confront and work through these volatile obstacles, they will become invaluable and effective tools that you will learn to use for personal and professional growth for better or for worse. Once these mines are diffused you can take them off of your plate and cast them aside as inert and harmless reminders of the lessons you will have learned along the way.

It is unbelievably refreshing when you can unload the baggage from the minefield that stood in your way of succeeding and may have been suppressing you into a defensive posture. It is a weight off your shoulders and the monkey is off your back — for now; then when he comes swinging back around you will know exactly what to do.

To employ mental toughness and fortitude you must find the primal instinct and visceral drive in your core to attack whatever may be forcing you to retreat from the line to establish a defensive rather than an offensive front.

Chapter 4

Availability, affability, & ability

Availability, affability, & ability:

the basic characteristics and

building blocks of a successful

house officer and physician.

Numerous attending physicians throughout the course of my training referred to the "three As" that constitute the basic characteristics and building blocks of a successful house officer and physician:

- Availability.
- Affability.
- Ability.

Let's dig a little deeper.

Availability:

You must make yourself available to participate in and maximize your own training. No one is going to do this for you. A strong work ethic cannot be taught nor forced. Every resident has to make themselves readily available to extract the maximum amount of value from their own training. The final product from your training will be a direct reflection of what you pour into it at the end of the day. If you put forth a lackluster effort, do not make yourself available, and do not exhibit a tireless work ethic, the end result will leave plenty to be desired.

You will see, if you have not already experienced this, some schmuck who will hide out in a call room, "accidentally turn off their pager," repeatedly bail out of work early, show up late, never volunteer to take on a project, or pull a myriad of other shenanigans to shirk their responsibilities because they are lazy

You must make yourself available to participate in and maximize your own training.

and their "give a shit factor" is indeed in the toilet. You can guarantee that these folks will be practicing medicine of inferior quality at the conclusion of their training if they make it that far.

Do not be a "yes-man," but make yourself available when opportunities for advancement, professional growth, and education come knocking on your cranium. Thank the others who do not have the drive that you possess for allowing you to step up to the plate and maximize your own training experience.

Affability:

This characteristic is not rocket surgery. We learned this lesson in kindergarten and it remains applicable to medical residents and surgical trainees. Nothing has changed here. Be easy to work with, get along with others, and be a team player. Be pleasant, professional, respectful, polite, and courteous. As sad as it may be, I feel that it is absolutely necessary to remind folks about this basic tenet of social etiquette as a plethora of residents seem to forget these values once they reach the level of a house officer.

I am not saying you need to be a cheerleader or a brown-noser. Please do not confuse being an overbearing ass-kisser with being affable. We have all seen these folks in action and there is nothing more nauseating.

Be easy to work with, get along

with others, and be a team

player. Be pleasant,

professional, respectful, polite,

and courteous.

A healthcare team that cannot collegially work together will ultimately fail and patient care will suffer as a result. If you are affable with your peers, attending staff, nurses, patient support staff, and patients, this simple act will pave the way for success. This simple and often overlooked fact truly cannot be understated.

I have witnessed humble, polite, courteous, and respectful house officers with an affable disposition, who may not be as smart, clinically savvy, or technically proficient as another star house officer, far exceed the performance of that star house officer who is rude, egotistical, entitled, and not a team player. Do not find yourself settling into the persona of the latter or you will find yourself wondering why you cannot seem to get ahead.

Ability:

You will notice that ability is the last of these three ingredients and it is the least important of the three. This may seem counter-intuitive but it is true. Even the most technically gifted surgeon or most intelligent clinician is severely handicapped if they do not make themselves available and if they are incapable of appropriately interacting with the healthcare team around them.

Even the most technically gifted surgeon or most intelligent clinician is severely handicapped if they do not make themselves available and if they are incapable of appropriately interacting with the healthcare team around them.

One can hone clinical acumen and technical prowess — ability; however, one absolutely cannot be taught a strong work ethic — availability, and you cannot force someone to be a team player — affability.

Take these characteristics to heart and live them every day throughout your training. It is truly a recipe for success.

Chapter 5

There is no substitute for experience

Without putting in the time you will not become the product you want to be nor your patients want you to be at the culmination of your training and beyond.

As noted in the last chapter, no individual is born an illustrious clinician or a technically gifted surgeon. Some residents may have a higher IQ than others and some residents may have a predilection to sound technical skills in the operating room compared with others. That alone is not what will make you successful. No one is born a savant diagnostician and no one in this world could expertly perform a Whipple procedure or fem-distal arterial bypass with a saphenous vein graft on day one of internship. These skills take years of experience to develop and the learning process will never end as the vast field of medicine expands at breakneck speed with new research, drugs, therapies, trials, and equipment hitting the scene every day.

Learning from your mistakes and maximizing your clinical experience is what will make you an outstanding clinician or surgeon. Without putting in the time you will not become the product you want to be or your patients want you to be at the culmination of your training and beyond.

Learning from your mistakes and maximizing your clinical experience is what will make you an outstanding clinician or surgeon.

Challenge yourself. Take the difficult cases and patients when others shy away. It will pay life-long dividends in your portfolio of professional development. In a culture dominated by work-hour restrictions, while this is important in its own right, the comprehensive training experience for resident physicians due to these restrictions has been somewhat diluted. There is a reason that medical and surgical training takes as long as it does to complete. You cannot become a competent clinician or surgeon overnight. It takes complete immersion, patient after patient, case after case, repetition after repetition, analyzing EKG after EKG, or reading CXR after CXR. You have to build the appropriate muscle memory and pattern recognition prowess particular to your specialty of choice and this takes time.

You cannot become a competent

clinician or surgeon overnight.

Do not take short cuts or you are putting yourself at a distinct disadvantage and you are putting your patients in danger. Neither is desirable and the latter is frankly unconscionable. Do not bail out of the operating room or ICU as you intensely watch the minute hand on the clock when your "shift is up." Stay in the operating room to complete the

Do not take short cuts or you are

putting yourself at a distinct

disadvantage and you are

putting your patients in danger.

operation you started or stay in house a little longer to ensure that the critically ill ICU patient you admitted is "tucked in" before leaving the hospital.

Doing things halfway does not do anyone any good. You need to be, and your patients need you to be, one-hundred percent engaged and in the game until the job is done. Maximize your clinical experiences and do not back down from the challenging patients you will inevitably run across. This will make you stronger, smarter, more confident, more capable, and more self-fulfilled to boot.

Despite the fact that you will have a senior resident, fellow, or attending physician hovering over your shoulder and watching you like a hawk as an intern or junior resident, you must challenge yourself to think independently about the patients you are seeing as early as possible in your training. Do not rely upon or allow your senior residents, fellows, or attendings to continuously spoon feed the appropriate information to you as you progress through a clinical scenario, procedure, or operation.

> *Do not rely upon or allow your senior residents, fellows, or attendings to continuously spoon feed the appropriate information to you as you progress through a clinical scenario, procedure, or operation.*

If possible, and it will not always be, due to patient acuity, extenuating circumstances, and other factors, ask senior colleagues who may be overseeing a case to allow you to present an independent plan of action or treatment plan first, no matter how simple the case may seem.

If a collegial relationship exists, politely interrupt the more senior folks you are working with when they launch into a diagnosis or treatment plan for a clinical scenario before you have had a chance to come up with an independently thought out plan of your own. Learn to independently analyze each clinical situation you come across and be prepared to present a course of action for whatever the scenario may call for. Come up with your own independent diagnostic assessment and plan regarding admission vs. discharge or continued observation, medication regimens, radiographic studies, appropriate laboratory studies, an operative approach, an operative maneuver, suture size and type, or a specific piece of equipment that may need to be employed in the operating theater depending on the clinical scenario you are working through.

Strive to stay one step ahead of any procedure or operation as it is moving forward and learn to be diligent in anticipating the next step of an operation or procedure. Be prepared to have a contingency plan for possible complications that may be encountered in a clinical scenario or surgical procedure. Learn to independently assess the clinical variables unfolding in front of you so that you can learn to make decisive decisions in real time.

Do not allow your senior residents, fellows, and attendings to constantly make these decisions for you. Learn to make decisions for yourself even if this is merely a mental exercise when no one really wants to hear what you have to say, which will be frequent as a junior house officer, while you are gaining

Learn to make decisions for yourself even if this is merely a mental exercise when no one really wants to hear what you have to say, which will be frequent as a junior house officer, while you are gaining your sea legs.

your sea legs. The more you put yourself through this type of mental exercise the more beneficial your training will be. You may regularly miss the mark as a junior resident as you are going through these independent learning exercises and that is okay. You are learning your craft and that is why you are there in the first place.

By independently assessing each situation on your own, patient after patient and case after case, without counting on the answers from your more experienced colleagues, you are building a massive cognitive database and enhancing your neuro muscle memory. You will gain tremendous benefit from this form of regular mental exercise compared with other house staff who coast along and may not participate in this critical independent learning opportunity.

Patients will decompensate and operations and procedures will find their way into trouble. The earlier in your training you can begin to critically problem solve and learn to think for yourself through a myriad of clinical situations, the more robust your training experience will be.

As you progress in your training you will be surprised that your own independent assessments will begin aligning with those of your seasoned senior residents, fellows, and attendings rather than missing the mark. Before long you will find yourself on your own without any back-up available and

The earlier in your training you can begin to critically problem solve and learn to think for yourself through a myriad of clinical situations, the more robust your training experience will be.

you will be thankful you challenged yourself in this way. Your experience will guide you during difficult cases and difficult times.

Experience is king!

Part II

HOW TO PLAY THE GAME

The most difficult thing is the decision to

act, the rest is merely tenacity.

Amelia Earhart

Chapter 6

Triage & preparation

There are no secrets to success.

It is the result of preparation,

hard work, and learning

from failure.

General Colin L. Powell

Throughout residency training you will constantly find yourself prioritizing and triaging a myriad of tasks twenty-four seven. The list of tasks will never end and sometimes it will feel like a torrential downpour of objectives to conquer. You will learn to master the art of triage not only in taking care of a large census of inpatients or multiple polytrauma patients in a busy trauma bay, but also in accomplishing the always present and unremitting administrative tasks that are ubiquitous throughout medicine. You will find yourself learning the craft of how to be in two places at once, how to grow an extra hand, and how to be tremendously efficient.

Throughout residency training you will constantly find yourself prioritizing and triaging a myriad of tasks twenty-four seven.

Of course, the most urgent patients or tasks will require your undivided attention first and foremost. This goes without saying. After you address these urgent or emergent issues it is then important to determine what small action items you can take off of your plate so you can then engage and attack a larger item that may consume a more significant amount of time and energy to complete.

Of course, the most urgent patients or tasks will require your undivided attention first and foremost.

By eliminating these smaller miscellaneous items and minutiae off of your to do list, you will have generated peace of mind by having them cleared away and you will not have these tasks vying for your attention or soaking up your thinly spread

By eliminating these smaller miscellaneous items and minutiae off of your to do list, you will have generated peace of mind.

bandwidth. It will allow you to focus on a larger task at hand, allow you to devote more attention and energy to a larger project, and make it that much easier to complete efficiently and expediently without undue distraction.

Another vital deliberate action that rivals the importance of proper triage during residency is preparation and planning ahead. You should constantly be considering what tasks you can accomplish ahead of time to make your next work day or next clinical activity run more smoothly.

Another vital deliberate action that rivals the importance of proper triage during residency is preparation and planning ahead.

Pilots often talk about, "staying ahead of the aircraft." Modern aircraft, especially tactical military fighter aircraft, can move at an incredible rate of speed. It is easy to fall behind in managing a supersonic aircraft due to the sheer speed that events are occurring. For the pilot there are a number of tasks that need to be completed in a timely manner, such as basic airmanship and maneuvers, navigation, communication inside and outside of the cockpit, and employment of weapon systems or other sensors. Pilots have to learn how to stay one step ahead at all times and this is no different than being a tremendously busy house officer. Learn how to stay ahead of the aircraft instead of it getting ahead of you. Learn to anticipate, prepare, plan ahead, and ultimately stay ahead of the power curve.

Get into the habit of reviewing your patient's charts on your inpatient service before leaving the hospital for the day and

Get into the habit of reviewing

your patient's charts on your

inpatient service before leaving

the hospital for the day and

review the list of office patients

you will see the next day if

applicable.

review the list of office patients you will see the next day if applicable. Most modern training institutions have electronic medical records making these tasks quite easy to execute from your desk, lounge, work room, or a work station in the ICU or ward. Ensure your inpatients have routine laboratory and radiographic studies ordered for the next morning if applicable and make sure any updates or changes to medications or therapies from the present day are appropriately reflected in your patients' order sets. This will prevent you from scrambling to play catch-up the next morning and prevent an attending or

Double check your patient's

vital signs, urine output,

consultant's notes, etc. at the

end of the day to be sure there

are not any acute physiologic

fires you need to put out before

leaving the hospital.

senior resident from breathing down your neck because labs or X-rays are not back in a timely manner during morning rounds. Also, double check your patient's vital signs, urine output, consultant's notes, etc. at the end of the day to be sure there are not any acute physiologic fires you need to put out before leaving the hospital.

Surprises will constantly spring up and more often than not it will feel like you are playing whack-a-mole as you put out fires, admit and discharge patients, answer pages, and field consults. You will develop your own algorithm to triage tasks and to stay prepared. Prioritize accordingly, prepare, check things off your list one by one in a systematic fashion, and things will get done efficiently.

Chapter 7

Delegate

You cannot do it all by yourself.

Even with a sound base of triage and preparation prowess you must also learn to delegate. You cannot go it alone and you cannot tackle it all by yourself; especially on a large inpatient service at a busy academic institution. There is just no way to get it all done on your own. Trust me, I have tried and I have failed miserably.

Most physicians have "type A personalities" and it is not easy for us to concede responsibility to others. You have to get used to letting some things out of your immediate control and let others share the load. Among the army of medical students, interns, residents, nurse practitioners, and physician's assistants on your team you can divide a lengthy list of tasks and conquer them in short order. All of these able bodies and

You must learn to delegate.

minds are force multipliers. Take advantage of the manpower on your patient care teams. This is how you will be able to move mountains. No one is going to expect you to carry the load all on your own. It is just not possible. Each person on your team, depending on their level of training and competence, has a role to play and tasks must be delegated to these individuals accordingly.

Each person on your team,

depending on their level of

training and competence, has a

role to play and tasks must be

delegated to these

individuals accordingly.

When you find yourself at the upper echelon of a patient care team as a senior resident or a chief resident do not forget to "trust but verify." This is especially true with your junior trainees on July 1st when a brand new crop of green interns hit the ward bright-eyed and bushy-tailed but also scared to death and with a lot to learn. Things should be double if not triple checked for accuracy and correctness. Once a good track record develops you can relax this "trust but verify" posture. However, remember to also practice "controlled paranoia" and make sure things are not only getting done correctly but that they are getting done correctly the first time around.

> *Things should be double if not triple checked for accuracy and correctness.*

Preach this point to your teams on rounds. "Do it right the first time." If it takes an extra minute to execute a task correctly the first time, do it. Otherwise you are going to waste more time, manpower, and energy righting a wrong that could have been prevented by taking an extra few minutes and making sure it was done correctly the first time.

"Do it right the first time."
If it takes an extra minute to
execute a task correctly the
first time, do it.

Chapter 8

Use the chain of command

Information is funneled, filtered, and acted upon appropriately as it ascends the chain of command so there are no key players left out of the equation and the upper echelons of your team do not get bogged down with information that may be effectively dealt with at lower levels.

In the military there is a strict "chain of command" in which information flows from one level to another. At the most basic level, information should flow from junior personnel up the ranks accordingly and ultimately ending with the most senior person in command.

At the most basic level,

information should flow from

junior personnel up the ranks

accordingly and ultimately

ending with the most senior

person in command.

A seaman recruit, who holds the lowest rank in the U.S. Navy, does not casually walk into a four-star admiral's office, who holds the highest rank in the U.S. Navy, and begin rattling off information at will. The admiral would either fall out of his chair laughing or have the poor seaman recruit swiftly thrown in the brig out of sheer rage. Per the chain of command, junior personnel feed information to an intermediate level of management who then pass the information to senior management.

The same goes for a medical team. For example, when working with a team of students, interns, residents, and fellows, the medical student does not personally seek out, call, or page the attending physician to notify them that a patient on their service has suffered an acute myocardial infarction. It is not the medical student's place to bypass the chain of command in this manner and directly engage the attending unbeknownst to the remainder of the team.

When this theoretical and misinformed medical student bypasses the interns, residents, and fellows, they are omitting extremely critical clinical information from the core medical care team who could react to this information appropriately and put an expedient and efficient plan of action into place as the information concomitantly ascends the chain of command.

Push information up the chain of command according to your level of seniority on the team you are working with. Information from the medical students should be shunted to the interns and junior residents, information from the interns and junior residents should flow to the chief residents or fellows, and then from the chief residents or fellows to the attendings.

Information from the medical

students should be shunted to

the interns and junior residents,

information from the interns

and junior residents should flow

to the chief residents or fellows,

and then from the chief residents

or fellows to the attendings.

As a junior resident if you think shirking this chain of command will "impress" your fellows or attendings because you are the one reporting a key piece of information hot off the press, you are dead wrong. Your attendings and your more senior colleagues will not appreciate this overture to bypass the chain of command. Disrupting the chain of command will require information to flow back down the chain in the opposite direction so that appropriate individuals can be informed and the appropriate actions can be taken. In the end this will waste time and energy for everyone. It may even delay appropriate actions being instituted and put patients at risk as a result of a delay in care.

As information flows up the chain of command, the majority of problems can usually be dealt with effectively or neutralized prior to reaching the top attending level. If Mrs. Smith needs a central line then this can usually be accomplished by one of the interns or residents. The fellows and attendings do not need to be involved in the majority of routine information that you funnel into the chain of command accordingly.

As information flows up the

chain of command, the majority

of problems can usually be dealt

with effectively or neutralized

prior to reaching the top

attending level.

By adhering to the chain of command, information flows in a step-wise manner as well as in an efficient and expedient manner. The chain of command allows information to be funneled, filtered, and acted upon appropriately as it ascends the chain. This prevents key players from being left out of the equation and protects the upper echelons of your team from getting bogged down with information that may be effectively dealt with at lower levels.

There are always exceptions to the rule; however, this is how business should typically be conducted via the "chain of command" for the large majority of day-to-day operations. It will keep you and your healthcare team out of trouble and on track by relaying information in an effective and expedient manner. Learn it, live it, love it.

Chapter 9

Ask for help

Primum non nocere.

~ First do no harm.

Some may tell you that as a resident, "Asking for help is a sign of weakness." This is merely an excuse for those who go around spouting this nonsense to puff out their chest and falsely inflate their own ego. The fact of the matter is if you hear someone saying that asking for help is a sign of weakness, it is just plain bullshit. If you find yourself in an uncomfortable situation or are unsure of the next safe step to take in a difficult patient care scenario, then asking for help is in reality a sign of maturity and good judgement.

I promise you that folks exalting, "Asking for help is a sign of weakness," have been there before too. They have asked for

If you find yourself in an uncomfortable situation or are unsure of the next safe step to take in a difficult patient care scenario, then asking for help is in reality a sign of maturity and good judgement.

help when they have had an "oh shit" or "pucker factor" moment and you will also. Do not fall into the trap of listening to whatever garbage they are verbally spewing. In reality they are flat-out lying.

Do not be afraid to say, "I don't know," or ask for help no matter what level of the training pipeline you find yourself. Even chief residents, fellows, and attendings for that matter find themselves asking for help from senior colleagues on a routine basis. It is expected, it is appropriate, and as I mentioned, it demonstrates sound judgement to know when you need to ask for assistance.

> *Even chief residents, fellows,*
>
> *and attendings find themselves*
>
> *asking for help from senior*
>
> *colleagues on a routine basis.*

If you find yourself in a position where you are uncomfortable, do not hesitate to call on a senior resident or attending for help. If they try to brush you off, demand they come to assist. After all, it is their license on the line. Load the boat with more experience and load it early before you find yourself up a creek without a paddle.

When summoned in the middle of the night your more senior colleagues or attendings will probably bitch and moan in a gravelly voice; however, do not let this dissuade you. Your senior resident, fellow, or attending will be grateful you called them when the dust settles. They would much rather you ask for help in getting bailed out of a tough situation than getting yourself and a patient into trouble.

Additionally, if a poor outcome occurs as a result of overextending your confidence or skill set, this will be an unpleasant surprise to your chief resident, fellow, or attending. And trust me, they do not like surprises.

> *If a poor outcome occurs as a result of overextending your confidence or skill set, this will be an unpleasant surprise to your chief resident, fellow, or attending.*

As you progress in your training and the more senior you become, the more independence you will be given in managing patients, performing procedures and operations, and making independent judgements. This does not mean you have the keys to the kingdom or that you can recklessly charge the attending's clinical credit cards with nefarious or risky clinical activities at will. You must still be cognizant of and recognize when you are pushing your limits of confidence and capability. Do not push a bad position and make it worse. Ask for help when you find yourself in a tight spot.

I am not saying you should call for help about every last little item that peaks your concern. You do not want to be the resident who constantly "cries wolf." If overall you are comfortable and confident working through a problem, then by all means plod on and get it done. When you find yourself unsure of which way to turn next or when that nervous pit in your stomach feeling becomes readily apparent, call in the cavalry before you push it too far.

You do not want to be the

resident who constantly

"cries wolf."

Remember the Hippocratic oath we all swore on day one of medical school as we donned our short white coats: "First do no harm."

Chapter 10

Avoid drama like the plague

You are not in residency to

enact the next series of

Grey's Anatomy.

No matter where you end up receiving your training you will encounter a medical student, intern, resident, fellow, or attending who gets themselves wrapped up into the web of a scandal, tawdry adulterous affair, contentious relationships with their peers, or substance abuse situation. DO NOT find yourself getting wrapped up into some idiotic situation like this. It will exhaust you mentally, physically, and emotionally which will leave zero effective time for you to actually be a house officer.

You are not in residency to enact the next series of *Grey's Anatomy*. Leave that up to the Hollywood actors and producers. You are in residency to become a board-certified physician in whatever field of medicine you choose to pursue. That is objective number one.

Getting yourself wrapped up in a drama-laden debacle is a recipe for disaster and unfortunately you will witness this more often than you think. When trainees find themselves tangled up in a web of drama, they are not doing themselves, their peers, their staff, their patients, nor their families any favors. Getting balled up into one of these dramatic misadventures is unnecessary and will do nothing more than stall your progression through residency training.

Getting yourself wrapped up in a drama-laden debacle is a recipe for disaster and unfortunately you will witness this more often than you think.

While you are busy putting the pieces back together from the carnage that has ensued from an idiotic situation you have found yourself tethered to, guess who will be taking on the extra load in your absence? Your peers and your colleagues. They will not be happy about it nor will your program director or chairman. If you think your innocent little escapade will be a secret, it will not. Everyone will know your business. Nurses, students, interns, residents, fellows, attendings, and support staff. EVERYONE. You may as well spell it out on your forehead.

Everyone will know

your business.

Do yourself a favor. Fly under the radar, stay out of the spotlight, avoid drama like the plague, be boring, keep your head down, and get to work. Do not bother yourself or get involved with needless gossip around the water fountain. We call this "scuttlebutt" in the Navy. This will not improve your clinical acumen on the wards, facilitate useful clinical or bench research, nor hone your technical prowess in the operating theater. You have better things to do and real projects to target your energy toward rather than getting involved with a bunch of dramatic mental floss. Do not waste your time and valuable bandwidth in this capacity.

Do yourself a favor.

Fly under the radar, stay out of

the spotlight, avoid drama like

the plague, be boring, keep your

head down, and get to work.

Contrary to popular belief, the gossip column is not a sound way to decompress. If you want to decompress go to the gym, go for a jog, go to church, or spend time with your family. Do not decompress by aimlessly gossiping about he said, she said, can you believe what she was wearing, can you believe he dumped her, or she slept with him, blah-blah-blah. Who cares! Do something useful with your time.

Residency will fly by if you take this approach in staying away from the drama that is always present among the background static. Filter it out. There will be plenty of it and you do not want any part of it.

Do you want to add more time to your training because you have found yourself in a tough situation that could have easily been avoided? Do you want to go through remediation due to

Residency will fly by if you take this approach in staying away from the drama that is always present among the background static. Filter it out.

the unnecessary amount of wasted time a really stupid decision or situation has produced and subsequently pulled you away from your clinical training? Be my guest and go have fun with that.

Chapter 11

Don't forget the administrative minutiae

The only things that are certain

in life are death, taxes,

and paperwork.

The administrative minutiae can be a silent killer. Be punctual and efficient in managing and completing the plethora of menial administrative tasks that comes along with medical training. There is no sense in bitching about it because that will not make it go away. You just have to grind through it and get it done. The only things that are certain in life are death, taxes, and paperwork.

This list of items includes but is not limited to: logging work hours, logging procedures or operative cases, staying current

Be punctual and efficient in

managing and completing the

plethora of menial

administrative tasks that comes

along with medical training.

on your medical licensure, and completing performance evaluations. Additionally, you will have patient records and charts to complete, such as discharge summaries, outpatient clinical notes, operative reports, etc.

In residency I personally developed the habit pattern of not leaving my office at the conclusion of every work day without logging that day's work hours or cases, completing that day's operative dictations or clinical notes, and cleaning out my e-mail inbox as well as replying to any e-mails that warranted a timely response. It was well worth every second of the extra time spent in getting these things cleared off of my desk. If you adhere to this rule you will never fall behind on all of the menial administrative tasks that will be competing for your valuable time.

Develop the habit pattern of not

leaving your office at the

conclusion of every work day

without logging that day's work

hours or cases, completing that

day's operative dictations or

clinical notes, and cleaning out

your e-mail inbox as well as

replying to any e-mails that

warrant a timely response.

Although you may spend an extra thirty minutes at the office, having these tasks completed and off of your work list will do wonders for your time management and peace of mind. This will not always be possible due to extenuating circumstances but if you can stick to this plan on a regular basis it will pay tremendous dividends in the long run.

Should you find yourself weeks, months, or yes, even years behind on some of these tasks you will never be able to catch up. I have seen residents fall prey to this. It is not pretty and it is completely avoidable. You will find yourself catching flak from multiple levels of your department including chief residents, directors, and maybe even the chairman of the department for your delinquencies. That extra few minutes taken every day to complete these menial administrative tasks will save hours and hours of mental pain and anguish.

The more you find yourself on "hit lists" for delinquent or incomplete administrative issues, the more you will begin to be cast in a negatively shaded spotlight among the higher administrative echelons of your program. You will start being referred to as "that guy" or "that gal" by your senior residents, directors, and chairman. If you couple being "that guy" or "that gal" administratively with poor clinical performance you will be setting yourself up for a cycle of utter disaster. Not only can you not "get your shit together" with your primary clinical job but you also "won't have your shit together" with the miserable but nonetheless necessary administrative minutiae.

Poor clinical performance coupled with poor administrative skills is a synergistic tornado of badness. It is like blood in the water for a school of hungry great white sharks off the

Australian Great Barrier Reef and the feeding frenzy will inevitably begin. Residents who repeatedly find themselves in this predicament will fall behind, receive poor evaluations, may find themselves remediating, or may even be dropped from a training program if egregious enough.

> *Poor clinical performance*
>
> *coupled with poor*
>
> *administrative skills is a*
>
> *synergistic tornado of badness.*

Bottom line: keep your administrative "shit together" and don't be "that guy" or "that gal." Spend the extra few minutes every day and get these things done before they become a

> *Bottom line: keep your*
>
> *administrative "shit together."*

serious problem if you fall behind. Being effective and punctual administratively is also a sign of being a professional.

The number of administrative tasks you will be responsible for will only increase with seniority as you ascend the residency training ladder, so get used to it.

Part III

PROFESSIONALISM

We have joined a "profession"

and you should strive to earn

the designation of a

"professional" every day.

Chapter 12

Professional appearance & behavior

Take pride in yourself, your appearance, and your behavior to professionally represent the field of medicine.

If you tell yourself that first impressions do not matter as an excuse to look sloppy at work then you are kidding yourself. Of course, first impressions, punctuality, and professionalism matter, especially in the profession of medicine as a physician.

To look like a professional you do not have to look like a marine in dress uniform on a recruiting poster every day but

First impressions, punctuality,

and professionalism matter,

especially in the profession of

medicine as a physician.

you do not want to look like a slob either. Take pride in yourself, your appearance, and your behavior to professionally represent the field of medicine.

There are no military regulations being exercised in civilian medicine; however, you should maintain a decent haircut and if you are a facial hair kind of guy then please keep your mane tamed to some degree. Wear clothes that are not ill-fitting and wear a decent looking clean white coat. I know as residents you do not make much money and time off can be scarce. Well, there are no excuses here. There will be enough money in the coffers and enough time off to get yourself a haircut, a shave, and reasonably priced clothes that fit well and look professional.

Avoid overly revealing or loud flashy clothing styles. And for the love of God, please do not wear a T-shirt to work.

Especially one with some quote spelled out on the front in big bold letters that you think is clever or funny. No one else will think it is cute or funny. Not only will you look immature and unprofessional but you will also draw negative attention to yourself.

Avoid overly revealing or loud flashy clothing styles. And for the love of God, please do not wear a T-shirt to work.

No one cares that you are trying to make a fashion statement or that you are a "rebel" or "wild child" by wearing a T-shirt with a quote bordering on inappropriate or with politically charged overtones. What self-respecting physician wears a T-shirt to work anyway? Put on a scrub top if you are wearing scrubs or wear professional attire if you are not wearing scrubs. We are professionals. We are not couch potatoes who can get away with wearing pajamas around the hospital looking like we just rolled out of bed to come to work.

Wearing scrubs is not an excuse to look like a slob. You still need to look professional.

Sure, they make medical fashion look funny, stylish, or cute on television, but that is not real life. We are not actors. You are not on the set of *Scrubs*, *Grey's Anatomy*, or *General Hospital* when you go to work. We are real physicians taking care of real patients. Your patients will draw a first impression and they want to know that they are being taken care of by a professional physician. Not some punk kid with a mohawk, neck and sleeve tattoos, facial piercings that make you look like a Christmas tree year-round, ear gauges, and a T-shirt that says, "EAT ME!" on the front. If you are into that look then more power to you but let's be honest, there is no place for that in the profession of medicine.

When your white coat begins to look like it is one continuous coffee stain that is fraying around the cuffs and collar, is threadbare, smells a little musty, and looks like it has been stuffed into a locker — get a new one. It should not be worn in this condition as a badge of honor signifying how hard you are working. We all work hard and no one cares. Get a new one.

Okay, it is five-o'clock in the morning in the ICU and you have been getting crushed with people trying to die on your watch all night. You are beat down and dragging ass. You will look haggard and a little sloppy. I get it. That is part of the deal sometimes. Just avoid sporting the run-down and haggard look

When your white coat begins to look like it is one continuous coffee stain that is fraying around the cuffs and collar, is threadbare, smells a little musty, and looks like it has been stuffed into a locker — get a new one.

all of the time. Try to get yourself cleaned up before morning rounds if possible. Sometimes it will not be possible and that is alright. Just do the best you can to maintain a professional appearance at all times and be punctual.

Multiple facets of professional behavior have been and will be further addressed so I will not belabor those points here; however, I wanted to bring up one additional point about professional communication and behavior at this juncture: profanity. There is a time and place for profanity to be used and it certainly does not include any occasion or location when there is direct patient care occurring. We all slip up from time to time and that is okay, but it should not be part of your regular repertoire with patients.

Save your shop talk, venting sessions, or frustrated exaltations for your private offices, private work spaces, or the bar down the street over a few cold ones. There is nothing wrong with that. This is fine anywhere other than public patient care areas in your outpatient clinics and hospitals as long as you are adhering to appropriate patient privacy principles. Blatantly speaking in profanities in front of your patients or within ear shot of your patients is unprofessional, indecent, and should not be tolerated.

Blatantly speaking in profanities in front of your patients or within ear shot of your patients is unprofessional, indecent, and should not be tolerated.

Chapter 13

Communication

Aviate, navigate, communicate.

Being a good communicator is an essential part of being a good house officer and physician. We discussed the "chain of command" already so I will not belabor that point. Inform your peers and the other members of your medical treatment team per the "chain of command" of any new information, problems, or developments in a timely, clear, and concise manner.

As a prior naval flight surgeon, I was fortunate to have proceeded through the same basic aviation training syllabus that all naval aviators progress through as they earn their "Wings of Gold." After completing basic flight training and subsequent aerospace medical training, I accrued flight hours in a number of different tactical fighter jet aircraft as an operational flight surgeon. One basic message was pervasive

Being a good communicator is

an essential part of being a good

house officer and physician.

and ubiquitous throughout the naval aviation community from the first days of aviation preflight training through to the complex operational missions and exercises in the fleet. Whether operating in the skies ashore or over open water from an aircraft carrier, the same basic mantra of executing safe aviation missions never changed, "Aviate, navigate, communicate."

The most important task a pilot must execute is to safely operate his airframe in the airspace he occupies or the airspace where he may be leading a flight of multiple aircraft. The second most important factor is to navigate effectively throughout the mission or "hop." You must maintain appropriate situational awareness at all times to know where you are going, how you are going to reach your objective, and how to return safely to your home air station or aircraft carrier at the conclusion of a hop. There is a big ocean out there and it is easy to get lost. Although a thousand-foot long aircraft carrier may seem like a massive piece of floating metal that would be hard to miss, it gets small in a hurry at thirty-thousand feet travelling at speeds in excess of Mach one.

After safely operating the aircraft and navigating appropriately, pilots and aircrew must thirdly in their echelon of priorities effectively communicate to maintain safe flight operations and to ensure mission success either in training flights or real world operational missions. Without effective communication, or when communication breaks down, operational risk management begins to decay exponentially, the potential for mission success degrades markedly, and the potential for an incident or devastating mishap increases significantly.

Effective, clear, concise, and expedient communication is one of the most important factors in the profession of medicine, as

Effective, clear, concise, and expedient communication is one of the most important factors in the profession of medicine.

it is in aviation. We can draw multiple parallels regarding the critical importance of effective communication as it pertains to medicine as well as aviation. A breakdown of effective communication in aviation as well as in medicine can transform a stable flight regime or stable patient into a situation that can rapidly deteriorate to chaos and spiral out of control. The stakes are high, possibly patients' lives, and all members of a medical team from top to bottom must maintain open lines of clear and effective communication at all times.

We live in a world of social media gone wild. Pagers have been taken over by smartphones and iDevices galore with text messaging and a myriad of other communication applications

We live in a world of social media gone wild...

Do not let these convenient and nifty methods of electronic communication get you into trouble.

such as Facebook, Twitter, Instagram, Snapchat, Facetime and the list goes on. Do not let these convenient and nifty methods of electronic communication get you into trouble.

"What do you mean?" you ask as you are checking the latest social media alert on your smartphone. "My new smartphone, and all the applications I have it loaded with, is the best thing since sliced bread," you say?

These applications and communication methods are fine for routine or non-clinical items if you and your healthcare team are on board using them. These methods of relaying information, however, are absolutely intolerable if there is time sensitive or highly important clinical information that needs to be distributed. The message may not go through on the application, the intended recipient's phone may be dead, they may sleep through the alert, their phone may be on silent mode, or they may be scrubbed into surgery or a procedure and unable to view the message in a timely manner.

Here's a novel idea: instead of using your messaging applications, dial their phone number and call them directly, or you could take a walk through the hospital to find the proper recipient of the information and talk to them like an actual human being. Unfortunately, these highly effective and quite simple methods of communication sometimes seem like a lost art when our world is so inundated with social media and alternative messaging applications.

Should you find yourself transmitting time sensitive or important information via text message or one of these applications on your smartphone, you must ensure a timely acknowledgement or response that this information was in fact received. If you do not receive acknowledgement then you

When time or the degree of

importance of clinical

information really matters,

forget the newfangled

smartphones and make sure

you actually see the desired

recipient of the information

face to face or you hear the

sound of their voice on the

other end of the phone line.

should never assume that the recipient actually acquired that message. In this case the next appropriate step is to make a phone call or put on your sneakers, get to stepping, and seek out that individual personally.

When time or the degree of importance of clinical information really matters, and it will on a regular basis as you care for critically ill patients, forget the newfangled smartphones and make sure you actually see the desired recipient of the information face to face or you hear the sound of their voice on the other end of the phone line.

If you have bad news to pass on, it should be communicated to the appropriate person in your "chain of command" in a timely manner and in no uncertain terms. Bad news only gets worse with time so do not try to perfume a pig by sugar coating bad news or omitting details. Lay it out as clear as day so that appropriate corrective action can be taken accordingly, efficiently, and expeditiously.

Good communication is one of the many key pillars to ensuring sound healthcare services.

Chapter 14

Integrity & character

Tell the truth for the

truth has no fear.

As a medical trainee you must work together with your peers, watch out for one another, and take care of one another through the inevitable peaks and valleys of your training. One team — one fight.

Do the right thing when no one is looking. Do not do a job halfway so your fellow residents have to pick up the pieces later when your half-ass job breaks down. Do not take the easy way out when you know the correct course of action, even if this is difficult. Tell the truth for the truth has no fear. This is integrity.

As a naval flight surgeon I developed a close relationship with the F/A-18 aviation squadrons I flew with and treated. In particular, I developed close relationships with the junior officers of those squadrons as I was a junior officer myself. The junior officers in the squadrons, or "JOs," referred to their collective presence and strength in numbers despite their junior rank as the Junior Officer Protection Agency or "JOPA."

The same goes for house officers who must stick together and watch each other's backs throughout the training process. Create a House Officer Protection Agency among yourselves and protect one another. If one of your colleagues is screwing something up or on the verge of getting themselves into trouble, recognize the folly that is looming and help them work their way out of the problem. If one of your colleagues is getting too big for their britches then knock them off their high horse and bring them back down to reality where they belong.

House officers must stick together and watch each other's backs throughout the training process.

If you make a mistake own up to it and never throw your colleagues under the bus. Tell the truth, take your licks, and move on. The more you try to hide a mistake, blame a mistake on someone else, sugar coat bad news, or delay bringing up bad news, things will only get worse for you when the truth comes to light. And after all, the truth always finds a way of coming to light, so do not run from it.

> *If you make a mistake own up to it and never throw your colleagues under the bus.*

As we have previously mentioned, do not let bad news be a surprise to your senior residents, fellows, or attendings. If something goes wrong, push the bad news out so that it can be dealt with accordingly. If you try to right a wrong as a means to make a bad situation better and avoid punitive consequences or otherwise, it is likely that you will do nothing more than make the situation worse. By simply relaying the bad news to the appropriate folks in your "chain of command" in a timely manner you will prevent a bad situation from spiraling out of control.

If something goes wrong, push

the bad news out so that it can

be dealt with accordingly.

Avoid the temptation to try and fix a problem that is well over your head without enlisting the help of your senior colleagues. It will likely lead to failure if you opt to take that road alone. If you do take this ill-advised road and escape unscathed you will be giving yourself a sense of false confidence that will likely lead to bigger troubles for you in the future.

Do not withhold information that would be beneficial to your fellow trainees for your own gain. Whatever you can do to

Do not withhold information

that would be beneficial to your

fellow trainees for your

own gain.

improve the lives of your colleagues, the better off your department will be and the happier your attendings, director, and chairman will be.

Although it may not seem like it at the time when you are in the process of having your rear-end chewed by senior residents, fellows, or attendings, these folks will truly not be disgruntled if you are trying your best and genuinely doing the best you can with the information and resources you have at your disposal in the event something unfavorable occurs. If they cannot recognize this then they are truly ass-holes and need to get a life.

Alternatively, if you are being lazy, found in direct dereliction of duty, found to be taking short cuts, or blatantly shirking your responsibilities, there will be no excuses and you will be dealt with swiftly, firmly, and accordingly. There is no place for a house officer or physician exhibiting this type of behavior. It will not be tolerated and you will unequivocally be asked to leave the profession of medicine if you engage in disingenuous behavior or demonstrate a lack of integrity.

Chapter 15

Check your ego at the door

You may be important but you are not as important as your ego wants you to be.

Do not act entitled because you are not. Be humble and have humility. You may be important but you are not as important as your ego wants you to be. If you think you are the smartest person in the room, chances are you are not, so do not go strutting around like a spring turkey thinking you are.

As soon as you begin to act egotistical and entitled you will be labeled as such with a scarlet E emblazoned on the front of your scrub top or white coat and usually looked upon with

> *Do not act entitled because*
>
> *you are not. Be humble*
>
> *and have humility.*

disdain from your peers and the healthcare team you are working with at large.

As physicians our "type A" selves have a healthy dose of ego and narcissism coursing through our veins. However, we are not full-blown egomaniacs and we do not typically carry a true "DSM" diagnosis of narcissism in our medical records. Sure, there are a few in every crowd but you must keep your ego healthily in check and do not become that egotistical and entitled house officer whom everyone despises. It will not do you any favors.

> *You must keep your ego*
>
> *healthily in check.*

Remember that while you are responsible for the majority of direct patient care and you work your tail off day in and day out, the real perception to everyone else is that you only comprise a small percentage share of the entire medical team that is actively caring for your patients. Among the patient care technicians, nurses, medical students, physician assistants, nurse practitioners, nutritionists, social workers, and other physicians, you are merely a blip on the radar in the grand scheme of things. This is particularly true in large academic centers. Although you may be carrying a heavy load of the patient care and you are working very hard, remember that you are not the end-all, be-all.

You will receive positive reinforcement, favorable evaluations, and personal accolades when warranted. For the time being, be humble and go about your work as a quiet professional.

Chapter 16

Arrogance, braggadocious, & the surgical dragon

You are only as good as

your last complication.

There are times in your training when it seems like you are sailing. Like Midas, everything you touch turns to gold, and you can do no wrong. Your performance academically and clinically is outstanding. Your patients are getting well, your staff is happy, and you are surfing on the clouds of medicine and surgery. You are untouchable.

Pinch yourself because you are dreaming. While these good times will occur on occasion, they will be short-lived and will come abruptly crashing down on top of you like a brittle house of cards in a matter of minutes. Be ready because it will happen. A rouge wave will come along, pummel you into the sand, and then wash you out to sea when you least expect it. It is not a matter of if, it is a matter of when.

The minute you become cocky, braggadocious, arrogant, or smug, the "surgical dragon" will seek you out and destroy you. Just when you are patting yourself on the back that a tough case went well, your patient is progressing without complication, and you prematurely celebrate, the fire-breathing surgical dragon will swoop down with fury and leave your lush green fields of contentment scorched to a smoldering crisp.

The minute you become cocky,

braggadocious, arrogant, or

smug, the "surgical dragon"

will seek you out and

destroy you.

Just when you are patting yourself on the back that a tough case went well, your patient is progressing without complication, and you prematurely celebrate, the fire-breathing surgical dragon will swoop down with fury and leave your lush green fields of contentment scorched to a smoldering crisp.

The Whipple that went so well now has an anastomotic leak and a gastroduodenal artery stump bleed requiring readmission to the ICU, transfusion, and interventional radiology angioembolization if not worse. That straightforward right hemicolectomy you crushed effectively curing the patient's low-stage colon adenocarcinoma now has an anastomotic leak and needs to go back to the operating room. Oh, and guess what else. The laparoscopic cholecystectomy you did five days ago is in the ED with a cystic duct stump leak that will also require IR intervention for percutaneous drainage of a biloma and endoscopic retrograde cholangiopancreatography with stent placement. Your pager startles you with two fresh consults in the ED too: an acute appendicitis and a high-grade small bowel obstruction that may need to go to the operating room. To top it all off, an alpha trauma alert, a gunshot wound to the chest, is about to hit the doors in the trauma bay.

Get the idea? Just when you think everything is rainbows and sunshine you will have an abrupt reality check hit you in the gut with the force of a freight train that will bring you scorching down from the outer earth orbit to sea level at atmospheric re-entry velocity. Remind yourself every day that you are only as good as your last complication. This little

Remind yourself every day that you are only as good as your last complication.

reminder will keep you humble and prevent you from falling into a falsely content temperament that will never last.

Never let your guard down. As a house officer your world can go from zero to the velocity of a ballistic missile in an instant. If you are not mentally prepared for situations like this because you are too busy patting yourself on the back it will throw you into a tail-spin that will be extremely difficult to recover from.

Never let your guard down.

I recall a particular case during my training that illustrates this point very well. I remember this case quite vividly and will not forget an invaluable lesson that I learned from it.

As a trauma chief resident at a busy level-one trauma center in the wee hours of a call shift I encountered a patient who rolled into the trauma bay with a stab wound to the precordium. He was severely acidotic, and hypotensive, with worsening cardiac tamponade and was literally on death's doorstep. Fortunately, this young patient had enough physiologic reserve to survive a quick trip from the trauma bay to the more controlled environment of the trauma operating suite. We rushed him into the trauma operating room, quickly performed a median sternotomy, evacuated a large volume of blood and clot from the pericardium, and repaired a penetrating injury to the right ventricle.

I followed the patient to the trauma ICU after the case and ensured all tubes, lines, drains, ventilator settings, medications, and various other sundry items were good to go. Once content with how the patient was doing and that all the details were buttoned up, I remember waltzing out of the patient's ICU room smiling from ear to ear and with a swagger in my step. As the adrenaline surge still lingered I was wholly satisfied with the surgery I had performed which had effectively snatched this dying patient away from the grim reaper's grasp.

One of the seasoned trauma attending surgeons was standing outside the ICU room at the nurses' station looking at me with a stoic and stern look as I emerged through the door. I will never forget what he told me. It stopped me dead in my tracks and provided me with a reality check like an open-handed slap to the face that I sorely needed.

He dryly said, "It's not a win unless he is sitting in bed eating a cheeseburger later tonight and walks out of here on his own in a couple of days."

It was a reality check and dose of humble pie that I sorely needed right then and there and I will never forget it. The patient ended up doing remarkably well but I had gotten way too far ahead of myself with the initial successes of an exciting trauma sternotomy and cardiac repair case which surgical residents can usually only dream about. I had no idea how this guy was going to do. He had a big operation, had narrowly escaped death, and there was a multitude of factors that could have turned this "great case" into a devastating one.

Remain humble, do not get ahead of yourself, remain vigilant, and always be ready for the worst. It will keep the

Remain humble, do not get

ahead of yourself, remain

vigilant, and always be ready for

the worst. It will keep the

surgical dragon at bay and it

will keep you operating on

an even keel.

surgical dragon at bay and it will keep you operating on an even keel.

Chapter 17

Roundsmanship

Practice "roundsmanship."

It is courteous, respectful, and it

is part of the learning process

for everyone.

As a house officer you will be responsible for running inpatient "rounds" at least once if not twice daily during the majority of your medical training. This is the classic time when the clinical questions start flying from the chief residents, fellows, and attendings, like darts in a smoky old pool room. Pointed clinical questions will be asked, typically to an individual, or sometimes to a group of individuals at a certain level of training such as the interns or junior residents.

Do not be the over eager ass-hole in the group who blurts out every answer to every question before the question can be finished. Practice "roundsmanship." It is courteous, respectful, and it is part of the learning process for everyone. Allow the person who was asked the question to answer the inquiry directly. If they do not know the answer, the individual asking the questions will typically help walk that person through the problem to a correct answer or they may open the floor for someone else to answer the question. At this point it is alright to chime in and demonstrate your clinical prowess.

Do not step on someone else's toes while they are fielding a question or scenario, especially someone senior to you. If the attending physician asks the chief resident or fellow a pointed question you definitely should not butt into their conversation as the junior resident, intern, or medical student and attempt to blurt out the answer. The attending was not asking you. They

Do not step on someone else's

toes while they are fielding a

question or scenario, especially

someone senior to you.

were asking the chief resident or fellow. This behavior will be frowned upon and will not be tolerated if you make a habit of it.

As you get closer to graduating from residency or fellowship, your board exams will be looming on the horizon. Frequently, the attending staff will begin prepping a senior resident or fellow for these examinations via a certain type of question or clinical scenario. Know your place. Let them work through this Q&A session at their level. This is not for you to get involved with as an intern or junior resident. Your time will come. Be quiet and soak it in. You will be surprised how much you can learn when you shut your mouth and open your ears.

You will be surprised how much you can learn when you shut your mouth and open your ears.

As a senior resident, chief resident, or fellow, your staff will sometimes clue you in on a particular topic of discussion for rounds. Alert your junior residents and medical students on the topic of choice for rounds so you can help them prepare and be ready. If they crush the attending's inquiries on rounds then you have also crushed it as a senior resident, chief resident, or fellow. This will be a direct reflection that you are teaching and you are getting your troops ready for combat. Kudos.

Chapter 18

The morbidity & mortality conference

What happens in M&M

stays in M&M.

During the course of residency training and beyond you will inevitably find yourself standing at a podium in the front of a room filled with medical students, interns, residents, fellows, and attendings discussing complications that have occurred involving a patient you have been caring for. An M&M conference may be more of a surgical-centric evolution; however, every medical specialty will have similar forums to discuss challenging or complex cases and the following discussion is applicable to all fields of medicine and surgery in that regard.

Intimidating as hell when you are a junior resident? Yes, but these presentations will get easier as you gain more experience. M&M presentations, or similar forums, as a resident are one of the more difficult things you will endure, but at the same time it is an excellent learning evolution. In time you will learn how to handle this like a pro.

> *M&M presentations, or similar forums, as a resident are one of the more difficult things you will endure, but at the same time it is an excellent learning evolution.*

Giving a solid M&M presentation is an art form in itself. Unfortunately, junior trainees typically learn how to do this through trial and error rather than frank instruction. Let's take a relatively deep dive into this process as it is an important one. Let's spend a little time on this topic, discuss a few key points to keep you on the right track, and try to prevent you from total derailment when you step up to the podium.

Initial rules of the road:

M&M conferences are not meant to be punitive although it sure seems that way sometimes. It is an important academic departmental conference, or even inter-departmental conference, so everyone can learn from the complications which have occurred and the laundry can be aired out. Things can get heated at times and there will be arguments and disagreements. That is the point. Let everyone air out what they need to say or voice any grievances if warranted. What happens in the M&M conference should stay in the room as an honor code principle.

M&M conferences are not meant to be punitive although it sure seems that way sometimes.

As you begin preparing for an M&M case presentation, remember that you need to be objective, be concise, and waste no time getting to the point. If you build a Powerpoint to assist

As you begin preparing for an

M&M case presentation,

remember that you need to be

objective, be concise, and waste

no time getting to the point.

with your presentation, keep the slide count to an absolute minimum and do not overload the slides with unnecessary details. Representative slices of cross-sectional imaging studies or plain films are helpful. You do not necessarily need to scroll through every slice of a CT scan or MRI. Keep it simple and to the point. Omit non-contributory and extraneous information.

Keep it simple and to the point.

Omit non-contributory and

extraneous information.

The M&M conference is not a place to be witty or make jokes. That is unprofessional behavior and will not be tolerated. It is not the place to be subjective, sugar coat problems, or try to perfume a pig as we previously alluded to when communicating bad news. Be objective, be frank, and get down to brass tacks without a bunch of fluff.

> *The M&M conference is not a*
>
> *place to be witty or make jokes.*

Preparation is paramount. Do your homework as you get ready for the presentation and be sure you have the details correct. Always discuss the case and review your presentation with the attending physician on record before you give your presentation. I cannot stress the importance of this enough. They will help you to hone the presentation and steer you away from trouble. They will help you correct key mistakes with your presentation or add in key details that you may have omitted to better frame the case during the presentation. You will both be on the same page prior to the presentation and this will avoid

> *Preparation is paramount.*

Always discuss the case and review your presentation with the attending physician on record before you give your presentation.

conflicting thoughts between you and your staff during the presentation, as well as avoid your staff from having to correct you during the presentation which never looks good for either party, especially for you as the resident.

First:

As you open up to present the case quickly, outline the patient's age, gender, diagnosis, procedure performed if applicable, the complication that occurred, and who your attending staff is for the case.

Second:

Provide a quick and concise patient history and physical examination as well as any pertinent laboratory and

Present the case quickly, outline

the patient's age, gender,

diagnosis, procedure performed

if applicable, the complication

that occurred, and who your

attending staff is for the case.

radiographic studies. This is not the time to regurgitate in exhausting detail the patient's non-contributory family history

Provide a quick and concise

patient history and physical

examination as well as any

pertinent laboratory and

radiographic studies.

dating back five generations, a ten-point negative review of systems, your head-to-toe physical examination, the MCV value and eosinophil count on the CBC, or a chest X-ray result from fifteen years ago. If there are pertinent positives and negatives, certainly mention them to frame your story appropriately. Including extraneous information will take up time and the gray-haired folks in the back of the room will begin anxiously shifting in their seats waiting for you to get to the point.

Third:

Outline the diagnosis of the patient and the treatment plan that was executed. Review the high points of any operation or operations that were performed, any key technical points, and any pertinent operative findings. You needn't recount every last detail of your incision length, every last millimeter of your dissection, or detail every last erythrocyte you blasted with your cautery stick.

> *Outline the diagnosis of the*
>
> *patient and the treatment plan*
>
> *that was executed.*

For example: "A laparoscopic appendectomy was performed under general anesthesia in the main operating room with standard infra-umbilical, left iliac fossa, and suprapubic midline port placement. Suppurative acute appendicitis was encountered with no evidence of gross perforation. Otherwise there were no other abnormal intra-operative findings. The mesoappendix was ligated and divided with a LigaSure™ energy device and the base of the appendix was ligated and divided with an Endo GIA™ 45mm stapler utilizing a blue tissue cartridge. The appendix was then extracted with an endoscopic retrieval bag from the infra-umbilical trocar site. The appendiceal stump staple line was interrogated and found to be intact and the divided edge of the mesoappendix was hemostatic. All trocars were removed and the port sites were then closed in standard fashion."

The intra-operative portion of your presentation is complete. Now move on. If the audience wants to know any additional information regarding the operation they will ask and you can politely oblige their request.

Fourth:

Present a concise postoperative course leading up to recognition of the complication that occurred. Again, keep this to the point with only the pertinent information required to

Present a concise postoperative

course leading up to recognition

of the complication that

occurred.

appropriately frame the story. No one cares what the patient's sodium level was on postoperative day number three. Hit the high points.

For example: "The patient developed an ileus and leukocytosis as well as recurrent febrile episodes and generalized abdominal pain with a large volume of pneumoperitoneum on plain films postoperative day number five status post-right hemicolectomy. This indicated an anastomotic leak and required an urgent return to the operating room for exploration. In preparation for operative exploration, the patient was resuscitated with crystalloid, intravenous antibiotics were started, and a type and cross-match was obtained."

There, you have hit the high points in one breath and painted a succinct picture without a long, serpiginous story that is difficult to follow. You will have outlined the clinical details of the complication that occurred and what diagnostics supported recognition of the complication as above.

Fifth:

You will discuss what intervention was performed as a result of the complication and how the patient ultimately progressed afterward.

> *Discuss what intervention was performed as a result of the complication and how the patient ultimately progressed afterward.*

Sixth:

Outline what you perceived to be the etiology of the complication. Was it a technical error at the index operation, the nature of the disease, an inappropriate diagnosis, a delay of diagnosis, etc.

Outline what you perceived to be

the etiology of the complication.

In conclusion:

You will complete your presentation with what you have learned from the complication at hand, what you would do differently in the future, how this complication has changed your practice pattern, and then offer to answer any questions.

Additional points:

More complex patients and more complex operations may warrant longer presentations, but regardless you should aim to be clear, concise, and avoid extraneous information that prolongs the presentation unnecessarily.

One key to honing your presentations is to project your voice so that everyone can hear you and do not rush yourself. Speak slowly enough so everyone can follow. This will avoid constant interruptions for you to repeat something and ultimately delay the presentation.

Use professional parlance and vocabulary instead of layman's terms for these presentations. Everyone in the room

Project your voice so that

everyone can hear you and do

not rush yourself.

should understand the specific lingo you are using and this will make for a more polished and professional presentation. If you use an abbreviation or acronym you better know what it means because you will be asked. Avoid slang and do not overuse unnecessary acronyms or abbreviations.

Use professional parlance and

vocabulary instead of layman's

terms for these presentations.

Do not say, "We did a lap chole with IOC because the LFTs were up." Instead, you should say, "We performed a laparoscopic cholecystectomy with intra-operative cholangiography due to elevation of the patient's transaminases and bilirubin preoperatively, as well as extrahepatic biliary ductal dilatation on ultrasonography concerning for possible choledocholithiasis."

Do not say, "We rolled back to the OR for a lap right hemi for cancer." Instead, you should say, "We performed a laparoscopic right hemicolectomy in the main operating room under general endotracheal anesthesia for biopsy proven and clinical stage one colonic adenocarcinoma."

Be objective. "The anastomosis kind of broke down." Nope, "The anastomosis leaked." Plain and simple language with no equivocation is what you are shooting for.

Be objective.

"The patient wasn't looking too good." Nope, "The patient began to clinically decompensate and develop signs of systemic embarrassment indicating an anastomotic leak and intra-abdominal sepsis." Much better.

"Kind of," "maybe," "a little bit," etc. should be stricken from your vocabulary for an M&M meeting and should be replaced with no uncertain objective terminology.

Take ownership of your mistakes

or the mistakes of the team even if

you were not at fault directly.

Take ownership of your mistakes or the mistakes of the team even if you were not at fault directly. This will happen from time to time. You were a member of the team, you are giving the presentation, and you need to take ownership of the complication as the resident at the podium. If you try to deflect the blame to someone else this is a recipe for disaster. If you try this you will begin a feeding frenzy of epic proportions from the senior staff in the back of the room. They do not want to hear it was not your fault. They want to hear what the problem was, what action was taken to fix it, how you learned from this complication, and they want to move on.

If you try to deflect the blame

to someone else this is a recipe

for disaster.

Defend your position and your decision-making process if warranted but never make excuses and never blame the patient. "The patient is a smoker and I believe that is why the anastomosis leaked." Nope, you screwed it up and it was a technical failure until proven otherwise. If you try to blame a patient for your technical error, error in judgement, or delay in your diagnosis you will be eaten alive and you will deserve it. Do not try to take the easy way out and blame the patient or someone else. Take ownership of the issue, get it over with, and move on.

Defend your position and your

decision-making process if

warranted but never make

excuses and never blame

the patient.

DO NOT RAMBLE! Do not stand up there and talk any more than you need to or you will begin to flail. Keep your presentation to the point and concise as we outlined above.

DO NOT RAMBLE!

Say what you need to say and SHUT UP! The longer you stand up there running your mouth the more off-the-cuff, ad-lib blunders you will make. The more you continue to ramble the more you will be bombarded with questions you did not prepare for, the dumber you will look, and the smaller you will feel. No one gets smarter at the M&M podium, especially as a junior resident. Do what you need to do and sit down.

Say, "I would," not "I could." No one wants to hear what you could do. The staff barking questions at the back of the room want to know what you would do when asked a pointed question about a clinical scenario. Choose a sound plan of action, defend your position, and be confident. If you are not sure what to do in a situation just say so. No harm no foul. That is one of the reasons you have found yourself at the podium. This is a learning evolution although at times it may feel a bit like being water boarded.

If you are not sure what to do in a situation just say so.

You will be asked how you would manage certain clinical situations or problems in the M&M conference, as well as on rounds and other academic teaching situations. In these situations the absolute last thing you want to do is make something up off the cuff that has never been published in a textbook. If you try this highly risky maneuver the seasoned staff in the back of the room will see right through you and you will nosedive into a spectacular ball of fire. The next thing you will see is your own blood leeching into the water and the sharks starting to school around you.

There may be staunch disagreements among the staff on how patients were managed during the course of your presentation. Unless you are a senior resident or fellow I would advise you to stay out of the argument at that point. Good job, you have tactfully maneuvered the primary focus of everyone's attention from you to the attending staff who are now verbally and academically duking it out among themselves. In this case just stand there and be quiet.

While M&M presentations are intimidating as a junior resident, they will become easier with experience and at the end of the day it is an excellent learning process. It will help you hone your public speaking skills, help you constructively learn from your mistakes, and it will help to prepare you for any oral board examinations that may be awaiting you at the end of your training.

There may be staunch disagreements among the staff on how patients were managed during the course of your presentation. Unless you are a senior resident or fellow I would advise you to stay out of the argument at that point.

We all must go through this as a rite of passage akin to the first days of medical school when we were thrust into the gross anatomy lab wide-eyed and apprehensive as hell. Take it in stride and learn from it. Your pride may get a little bruised and bloodied but you will survive and it will make you smarter, more resilient, and stronger.

Part IV

TALKING TO
PATIENTS & FAMILIES

I've learned that people will forget what

you said, people will forget what you did,

but people will never forget how you

made them feel.

Maya Angelou

Chapter 19

Lay it out in layman's terms

If you go around talking to
patients spouting medical
parlance that only your
colleagues can understand, your
patients are going to look at you
like you have three heads.

It goes without saying, but is important for us to remember, that as we have complex clinical conversations with our patients we must speak to our patients and their families in plain layman's terms.

We must speak to our patients

and their families in plain

layman's terms.

If you go around talking to patients spouting medical parlance that only your colleagues can understand, your patients are going to look at you like you have three heads. Slow down and break it down so your patients can understand. Speak in plain and easy to understand terms. If you do not take this approach then one of your fellow residents, fellows, or attendings are going to have to go through the whole conversation again.

It is perfectly acceptable to use the proper medical verbiage as long as you also tell your patients the appropriate layman's terms either before or after you rattle off the medical jargon.

I have found it helpful to draw basic pictures or diagrams, explain basic anatomical figures from a patient brochure or textbook, or even review graphics from the internet. A picture is sometimes worth a thousand words. It cuts to the point and patients can more easily relate to this. It will save time for you and will be tremendously helpful for your patient's understanding.

It can be helpful to draw basic pictures or diagrams, explain basic anatomical figures from a patient brochure or textbook, or even review graphics from the internet.

An example of what not to do:

Resident Jones: "Ma'am, you have a pheochromocytoma that is secreting excess metanephrines into the bloodstream causing episodic headaches, diaphoresis, and hypertension. You will require an adrenalectomy for this after we treat you with an alpha-blocker and beta-blocker to control your hypertension and tachycardia."

Mrs. Smith: "Huh? What! Could you speak English please? I am terribly confused."

143

A better way to tackle this:

Resident Jones: "Mrs. Smith. You have a tumor on your adrenal gland that could be a cancer. This will require us to treat you with some medications to control your heart rate and blood pressure followed by removal of your adrenal gland with surgery and it will need further testing to determine if it is cancerous. The adrenal gland is a small lump of tissue that sits on top of your kidney and secretes different hormones into the bloodstream. This tumor is producing excess levels of adrenaline. Adrenaline is the chemical that makes your heart race and your breathing quicken when something scares you. The adrenaline is going into your bloodstream and is causing your symptoms of headache, sweating, and high blood pressure. This tumor is called a pheochromocytoma. It is a difficult word to say and even more difficult to remember. Here is a print-out with the name clearly written, some additional information, and some pictures to help you understand what is going on. Let's take a few minutes to review this and I will be happy to answer any questions you may have."

You have summed up the clinical situation clearly, succinctly, and in relatively short order. Give your patients a moment to process what you have just told them and allow them to ask questions. We will delve more into this in the next chapter.

Give your patients a moment to process what you have just told them and allow them to ask questions.

Chapter 20

Delivering bad news

When speaking to a patient or a

family about death or a

diagnosis with a poor prognosis,

be empathetic but also be

objective and be direct.

If you have not had the experience of personally breaking difficult news to a patient or a family in medical school, you will definitely experience this at some point during your residency training.

When speaking to a patient or a family about death or a diagnosis with a poor prognosis, be empathetic but also be objective and be direct. Do not be misleading and do not try to sugar coat the bad news as this will give mixed signals that may confuse them. Do not beat around the bush. Say what needs to be said in no uncertain terms and then be quiet.

If a patient has died you must tell the family just that: "I am sorry to be the one to tell you this news but your father has died." Not "expired" or "passed" but "died" or "dead."

If a patient has cancer you must tell them just that: "I am sorry to be the one to tell you this but you have cancer." Not a "tumor," "lesion," "malignancy," "growth," or "neoplasm" but "cancer."

If this seems insensitive, it is not. You are being open and honest in no uncertain terms. What would be insensitive is to beat around the bush so the patient or family is receiving mixed signals and is not exactly sure of what is actually happening.

Give them a moment to begin processing the information and then politely ask if they have any questions. The sudden news of death or cancer will stop anyone in their tracks. After you say the words death or cancer to a patient or their family, they will not hear much else after that.

Give them a moment to begin

processing the information and

then politely ask if they have

any questions.

Let's go through a few scenarios here to illustrate and provide some helpful pointers on how to address these challenging conversations.

Starting the conversation:

If it is unclear what a patient or their family has or has not been told regarding a particular diagnosis or outcome, an easy way to begin the conversation is as follows:

"Tell me what you understand about your diagnosis or what the current situation is at this point."

Allow them to tell you what they know and you will get an idea of how you need to proceed next.

Scenario #1:

If a patient says:

"I've been told I have a breast cancer."

At this point they have already received the initial shock of the cancer diagnosis and you can proceed accordingly with the conversation.

Scenario #2:

Alternatively, if a patient says:

"They told me I need to come to the office today to talk about my biopsy results."

You now need to begin the conversation with explaining the diagnosis in no uncertain terms first as we outlined above and then proceed stepwise from there.

"Yes, Mrs. Smith, that is correct. I am sorry to be the one to deliver this news to you but your biopsy results have confirmed that you have breast cancer."

In this case you have provided the news about the cancer diagnosis succinctly and in no uncertain terms. Allow them to process the news, allow them to ask questions, and then move on accordingly.

Concluding the conversation:

An effective way to end a difficult conversation is to tell the patient and their family if present, "You will have a million questions that will come up before we speak again. I would like for you to please write them down so you don't forget them and I can answer them for you later."

If a patient or family is trying to ask you a lengthy list of questions you may not have time to answer them all due to more urgent clinical responsibilities. There may be more pressing issues for you to address and that is alright. A good way to deal with this situation is to politely tell them you are tending to an emergent or urgent patient matter and you or a colleague will return as soon as able to sit down with them and answer any and all questions they may have without interruption.

If you are unsure of the answer to a question a patient or a family member may have, then do not make something up. Let them know that you do not know the answer to that specific question but you will find out from a senior colleague or an attending and you will get back to them with the answer as soon as possible.

If you are unsure of the answer

to a question a patient or a

family member may have, then

do not make something up.

Chapter 21

Empathy

Empathy is not just an emotion

or an act. It is a gift you are

giving as a caregiver to your

patients or their family

members when they

need it most.

If you have not already, at some point you will sit at the bedside of a patient who is slipping from the bounds of life when there is nothing more that can be done to save them. You will be with the family members as their loved one passes from

You will be with the family members as their loved one passes from the living world and they will at times turn to you for comfort, a shoulder to grieve on, or even guidance.

the living world and they will at times turn to you for comfort, a shoulder to grieve on, or even guidance.

Be there for them. Hold their hand, pray with them, and embrace them if you are comfortable doing so. All will be appreciative of your efforts to care for the patient as well as the loved ones surrounding the patient during these difficult and emotional times.

Go the extra mile. Get a cup of coffee or a blanket for the family members. Offer to page the chaplain on call for them. You do not do these things because it impresses your attendings. You do these things because you are a human being

Be there for them. Hold their

hand, pray with them, and

embrace them if you are

comfortable doing so.

too. You have real emotions and real feelings like everyone else. Remember that.

Sometimes in medicine and surgery we are taught to be cold, flat, apathetic, detached, and stoic. We are taught to compartmentalize our emotions and feelings. Do not allow yourself to become a cold and emotionally detached physician. Most of us joined the profession and service of medicine to allay pathology, disease, illness, injury, and suffering. If you lose this empathetic drive then you will no longer gain true satisfaction that the practice of medicine and surgery has to offer. Maintain the passion in your heart and soul to care, to heal, and to ease the pain your patients and their family members are suffering through.

Empathy is not just an emotion or an act. It is a gift you are giving as a caregiver to your patients or their family members when they need it most.

Do not allow yourself to become

a cold and emotionally

detached physician.

Part V

PROVIDER WELLNESS

If you don't take care of yourself you won't be able to care for others.

This following section regarding provider wellness is not meant to be a medical or mental health text. If you are reading this you are probably a physician and have a commanding knowledge of these subjects that far surpasses the extent and purpose of this text.

This brief portion of the book is meant to be a reminder that these subjects should not be ignored during your training. These are not textbook chapters about nutrition, sleep physiology, or exercise physiology; however, these are subjects that should be kept at the forefront of your mind in promoting

There is no question that the stress and commitment required to progress through residency takes its toll on your health. You can combat some of these ill toward effects with a little bit of willpower and effort.

your own provider wellbeing throughout your training. You will need it. And after all, if you do not take care of yourself you will not be able to care for others.

We all know physicians make the worst patients. Adhering to these provider wellness principles during a busy and challenging residency is easier said than done but it is tremendously important. I implore you to take this to heart. I certainly wish that I would have been more ardent about maintaining a healthier lifestyle throughout my training. It will make a tremendous difference in your residency experience, help you perform at a higher level, and provide more satisfaction throughout the course of your training.

We have all seen interns who begin residency thin, fit, bright-eyed, energetic, with uncorrected twenty-twenty vision, and with plenty of hair who emerge from the other end of training overweight, worn-out, myopic, and bald.

There is no question that the stress and commitment required to progress through residency takes its toll on your health. You can combat some of these ill toward effects with a little bit of willpower and effort. Now get to it.

Chapter 22

Nutrition

You are what you eat.

As a previous surgical resident I lived on burned coffee, stale Graham crackers, and Ensure® nutrition shakes pilfered from the ICU between surgical cases and throughout long hours of in-house call as well as potato chips and candy bars from the hospital gift store. Obviously, this was not a great nutrition plan to fuel five years of grueling surgical training. I certainly did not do myself any favors with this abominable approach to fueling my mind and body.

I gained weight, became slow, and was constantly fatigued. I was always ravenously hungry and overall did not feel well. This in large part was due to poor nutrition throughout the majority of my training.

While high fat and carbohydrate laden foods will push you through in a pinch and light off the dopamine pleasure centers in your brain to bathe in that feel-good neurotransmitter for the short term, the crash is looming on the other side. When the crash comes it will leave you feeling flat and deflated.

Keep healthy snacks in a lounge, call room, office, nurses' station, or anywhere else that is readily accessible. Calorie dense and high carbohydrate foodstuffs will give you a jolt of energy albeit one that is not sustainable. Sources of nutrition with lean protein, fiber, healthy fats, and high water content are what you need to maintain a source of steady fuel that is satiating and won't produce a surge followed by a crash.

Keep healthy snacks in a lounge, call room, office, nurses' station, or anywhere else that is readily accessible.

Do your absolute best to eat three relatively balanced and healthy meals a day. Easier said than done, I know. Skipping

Do your absolute best to eat

three relatively balanced and

healthy meals a day.

meals will only produce a moody and insatiable beast that will overconsume and make poor nutritional choices when you do get the chance to belly up to the dinner table. After you glut yourself, when you do get the chance to eat you will then find yourself in a postprandial comatose state with a brain-gut circulation shunt occurring. You will feel tired, slow, and even more run-down as a result.

Another important thing to remember is to drink plenty of water. Caffeine is a must, I get it, but avoid overloading yourself with coffee, soft drinks, or those highly marketed supercharged energy drinks. The crash on the backside from these products

Another important thing to

remember is to drink

plenty of water.

will be waiting for you. Water will keep you well hydrated, keep you from feeling ravenous and voraciously hungry, and it will keep you performing at your best.

Maintaining a decent diet with wholesome nutritious foods during residency will keep your mind and body running at optimal levels. You will feel better, you will perform better, and your body will thank you for it at the conclusion of your training.

Chapter 23

Exercise

If all you can seem to do

somedays is take the stairs

instead of the elevator, do it.

Whatever you can do is better

than nothing.

For most individuals, residency is not the time to become a world-class triathlete or body builder; however, you should strive to partake in at least a small amount of physical exercise three to four times per week as able. This does not have to be an all-out, steroid fueled, protein shake guzzling, push yourself to total exhaustion workout session.

You should strive to partake in

at least a small amount of

physical exercise three to four

times per week as able.

If you have the opportunity to perform twenty to thirty minutes of cardiovascular aerobic conditioning a few days per week and mix in resistance training a few days per week, that is a great place to start. Resistance training does not require a weight bench or a myriad of expensive exercise machines. If you have access to this, great, but if not, push-ups, pull-ups, body weight squats, burpees, and sit-ups for strength training in an office or call room is a great alternative and is really all you need.

You do not even need to bother with a gym membership to execute this basic physical training plan. If you want to have a gym membership or do more physical training then by all means have it. That is fantastic; go for it.

When times are busy and time off is scarce, every little bit helps. If all you can seem to do some days is take the stairs instead of the elevator, do it. Whatever you can do is better than nothing. Do not be discouraged if you miss a week here or there because you are otherwise engaged in pressing clinical duties. Jump back in when you can and do not give those missed days another thought.

If you have the opportunity to perform twenty to thirty minutes of cardiovascular aerobic conditioning a few days per week and mix in resistance training a few days per week, that is a great place to start.

You will likely not be at peak physical condition during your medical training although any effort to partake in regular physical training or exercise will help you stay fit, focused, and confident. Physical activity will produce a surge of endorphins pumping through your blood stream which will be uplifting and it is a great way to clear your head as well.

Chapter 24

Sleep

Falling too far behind on your

sleep debt can at times leave you

wandering around the wards

like a zombie with just enough

functioning brain power

to be dangerous.

This topic speaks for itself so we will not belabor this point too much here.

You absolutely must sleep when you can. Restorative sleep to re-energize and refresh is paramount to performing at your best during medical training. A good night of restorative sleep to chisel away at your inevitably accruing sleep debt, that is constantly tumbling and plunging into red figures during residency, will do wonders for your attitude, performance, and temperament.

Restorative sleep to re-energize and refresh is paramount to performing at your best during medical training.

Capitalize on extra sleep whenever possible: weekends, holidays, time off, vacations, or whenever these opportunities arise. Whenever possible, silence your phone and pager while off duty so you can avoid unnecessary distractions that will only further interrupt your sleep cycle.

Periods of sleep facilitated by too much alcohol is not the same as real restorative sleep, so do not count a period of rest after a night of decompressing over one too many cocktails as real restorative sleep.

Periods of sleep facilitated by too much alcohol is not the same as real restorative sleep.

Sometimes you will have to forego other enticing social events or extracurricular activities to rest your mind and body. At times you will need to triage and sacrifice attending an exciting social or extracurricular non-work-related event in lieu of getting some sleep.

I cannot stress the importance of getting adequate rest or catching up on rest whenever possible during residency. Your sleep-wake cycle will be chaotic enough as it is with different shifts, long hours, and overnight in-house call. Mitigate the negative effects on your sleep-wake cycle as often as possible by catching up on your sleep debt.

Sometimes you will have to forego other enticing social events or extracurricular activities to rest your mind and body.

Falling too far behind on your sleep debt can at times leave you wandering around the wards like a zombie with just enough functioning brain power to be dangerous. Eat when you can and sleep when you can.

Chapter 25

Work hard, play hard, & better living through chemistry?

Drugs and alcohol can be an escape and a safe haven for medical trainees to turn to. Let's face it, residency is exceedingly stressful and sometimes it stings. As much as drugs and alcohol can soothe that sting, it is an enormously unhealthy and toxic way to cope with the stressors of your training.

There is no question that in residency you will work unbelievably hard and you will need time to let your hair down, decompress, and to blow off steam. You should absolutely do this as frequently as the opportunity presents itself.

In residency you will work

unbelievably hard and you will

need time to let your hair down,

decompress, and to blow off

steam.

Spend time with your family and friends, exercise, go to church, play sports, play golf, play tennis, go flying, go hunting, go fishing, go scuba diving, go shopping, watch movies, paint, or read. Read something other than medical texts please! Do whatever you can to clear your mind and not think about work or medicine for a while. It will do wonders for your health, mind, and spirit. It is refreshing to leave it all behind for a while and you will need to do this on a regular basis to cool your jets, recharge your batteries, refuel the tanks, and to mitigate burnout.

Spend time with your family

and friends, exercise, go to

church, play sports, play golf,

play tennis, go flying, go

hunting, go fishing, go scuba

diving, go shopping, watch

movies, paint, or read. Read

something other than medical

texts please!

You will be burning the candle at both ends with work alone. Do not try to light another candle with social excesses during your training. As with all the great things in life, including decompression from work with a few cocktails, partying, or drinks at your local watering hole, all things in moderation is key. It will be important and healthy for you to loosen up and decompress with your peers. It will be important to vent, lament, and commiserate about your training with your comrades over a few drinks and you absolutely should if you are so inclined to imbibe in a few adult beverages. However, be aware of your alcohol consumption and also that of your peers.

Drugs and alcohol can be an escape and a safe haven for medical trainees to turn to. Let's face it, residency is exceedingly stressful and sometimes it stings. As much as drugs and alcohol can soothe that sting, it is an enormously unhealthy and toxic way to cope with the stressors of your training.

Be self-aware and be honest with yourself if you feel like you are slipping down the slope of an alcohol or drug abuse

Be self-aware and be honest with yourself if you feel like you are slipping down the slope of an alcohol or drug abuse problem as a way to cope with your training and seek help immediately.

problem as a way to cope with your training and seek help immediately. Moreover, watch out for your comrades. I have unfortunately seen first-hand the carnage and resultant fallout of alcohol abuse as well as the negative impact of it upon the career and lives of medical residents and their families. It is not pretty. In fact, it is ugly, it is sad, and it is not easy for them to recover from if they can recover at all.

If you see a fellow trainee falling prey to the addiction and abuse of drugs or alcohol, you must intervene. Do not ignore this problem or pretend it will go away. If you turn a blind eye you are just as much at fault. It will not be easy to intervene but you must and you must not delay. Those who have fallen into an alcohol or drug abuse problem are putting themselves, your patients, and your institution at risk for a catastrophe.

If you see a fellow trainee falling prey to the addiction and abuse of drugs or alcohol, you must intervene.

You must seek out assistance and guidance to prevent harm to your fellow trainees, your peers, your patients, and others that may get caught in the crossfire along the way. Do not take no for an answer in the event you engage your colleagues, chief residents, fellows, program director, or even your chairman if they want to ignore the facts, turn a blind eye, or sweep things under a rug when you confront them regarding someone you are concerned about has a substance abuse problem.

You must seek out assistance and guidance to prevent harm to your fellow trainees, your peers, your patients, and others that may get caught in the crossfire along the way.

This would be the time to supersede your chain of command and do not stop knocking on doors until someone will listen to you and help you intervene. I have seen multiple echelons of leadership sweep these issues under a rug or assume a resident with a suspected substance abuse problem will work itself out. If it is truly a problem it will not simply fizzle out. Sooner or later there will be a major adverse event that could have major accompanying legal implications or the individual will hit absolute rock bottom and may be too far gone to help at that point.

I have seen residents get charged with DUIs and be admitted to the hospital in delirium tremens from alcohol withdrawal. It is not a pretty sight. The warning signs were there and action unfortunately was not taken until it was too late. Some can recover and some cannot. Act before it is too late. Sometimes having the guts to do the hard thing is absolutely the right thing to do. Find a way to get these folks some help before the damage is done and is irreparable.

Chapter 26

Physician burnout

Burnout in itself is not the problem; however, lack of recognition or admission of a burnout situation is what will get you into trouble.

You will go through periods of physician burnout. The bottom line, you will, and that is okay. It demonstrates sound introspective personal recognition when you identify that this is occurring. No harm, no foul. Take a step back, slow down, collect yourself, and do what you need to do to get going again.

You will go through periods of

physician burnout.

Burnout in itself is not the problem; however, lack of recognition or admission of a burnout situation is what will get you into trouble.

Take a step back, slow down,

collect yourself, and do what you

need to do to get going again.

It is okay to emotionally break down or burn out as long as you can put it behind you with the appropriate action and then light the torch again. When the stress of your medical training is coupled with other stressors life throws your way, even the most stoic of individuals can become overwhelmed. Take some time to decompress, get it out of your system, and it will be a weight lifted off of your shoulders. You can shake it off and get back into the saddle. Jettisoning whatever emotional baggage

It is okay to emotionally break down or burn out as long as you can put it behind you with the appropriate action and then light the torch again.

may be dragging you down will be refreshing and it will give you a fresh outlook to start anew.

When you have periods of burnout, be frank, open, and honest about it with yourself, your chief residents, and your program director. Maybe you just need a few days off to work through some personal problems or otherwise. I ensure you that your chain of command would rather you let them know what is happening in your life and work, and enable you to take some time off to get through the situation. If you ignore a true developing burnout situation and you push yourself to keep revving to the red line without intervention, you will reach a point where you are mentally, physically, and spiritually incapacitated. At that point a lengthy recovery may be required when you could have thwarted a major meltdown earlier on.

When you have periods of

burnout, be frank, open, and

honest about it with yourself,

your chief residents, and your

program director.

There are numerous resources for trainees to turn to when feeling burned out and I would encourage you to seek out these resources if you find yourself in this situation. Turn to a mentor, your chief residents, your program director, a chaplain, or your institutional provider wellness committee for help.

The important thing here is to recognize you are flaming out, admit to it, and deliberately take some effective action to stay ahead of it. When a fighter pilot's jet engine flames out he does not wait until he is out of airspeed and altitude, a.k.a. a crash, to do something about it. He takes appropriate action before the situation spirals out of control to get himself out of a bad situation. If the engine will not restart while airborne or if there is no airfield nearby to commence an emergency landing, this may require the pilot to eject or bail out. It's better to lose the aircraft than both the aircraft and the pilot. A price can be put

Turn to a mentor, your chief residents, your program director, a chaplain, or your institutional provider wellness committee for help.

on an aircraft and new ones can be built. The same does not go for the pilot if he goes down with the plane when he had the chance to have bailed out safely.

Get ahead of a burnout situation when you feel it looming. Do not try to ride it out and end up going down with the ship.

Part VI

FAMILY, FRIENDS, & FINANCES

A truly rich man is one whose children

run into his arms when his hands

are empty.

Unknown

Chapter 27

Family & friends

You will make sacrifices throughout your training and your family will also make deep sacrifices during your training as they stand by your side to support you through the process.

Ensure your family members and close friends are well aware of the time commitment and dedication that will be required to devote to your training before it begins. Most folks who are not in the business of medicine understand the training process and work hours of residency to be significant; however, they typically do not truly understand the sheer magnitude of the time commitment that is required.

Ensure your family members and close friends are well aware of the time commitment and dedication that will be required to devote to your training before it begins.

If you are married or in a serious relationship I would encourage you to talk to a couple who has lived through and successfully survived the residency training experience. Divorces, separations, and marital problems are a very real thing for couples going through medical training. It is stressful, the time commitment is vast, and it takes hard work to maintain a healthy marital or serious relationship throughout the training process.

Your family and significant others deserve to know what you will be getting yourself and them into. It is not fair to keep them in the dark and allow the reality of the time commitment to be a surprise once you get started. Provide a realistic mental framework of your day to day and long-term training schedule for your spouse, significant other, children, and other family members before you begin training. This will mitigate numerous conflicts once you are deeply entrenched in your training and prevent many unnecessary arguments.

Every resident has to work out their own personal balance of work and family time as they progress through their training.

Every resident has to work out their own personal balance of work and family time as they progress through their training.

While a resident has to be driven, focused, and wholeheartedly engaged in their training, this operational tempo cannot be sustained twenty-four hours a day, seven days a week, for years on end. Everyone needs a break. You will need a break and moreover your family will need a break from the grind as well. Give yourself a break and give your family a break too. You deserve it and they deserve it. You will miss them and more importantly they will miss you.

You will make sacrifices throughout your training and your family will also make deep sacrifices during your training as they stand by your side to support you through the process. Do

Everyone needs a break. You will need a break and moreover your family will need a break from the grind as well. Give yourself a break and give your family a break too. You deserve it and they deserve it.

not forget that they are at times suffering through this with you. This is a team sport when you have a family involved.

Your spouse, children, and other family members that may be living with you will keep the home fires burning while you are progressing through your training. For this they deserve tremendous credit, adoration, and respect. It is not easy for them either. The long hours, the long shifts, the long call nights, working weekends and holidays, calls in the middle of the night, and all of the other surprises that will come up along the way will take their toll. Remind them often how much you appreciate their support and that it would not be possible without them.

Remind your family often how much you appreciate their support and that it would not be possible without them.

You will be allotted a certain number of vacation days each year. My advice is to use all of them; plain and simple. Take a vacation with your family or have a stay at home vacation if that suits you better. I do not care what you do but take a break and give your family a break as well.

If you push and push without taking a break, which is tempting for our "type A" personalities, it will catch up with you and your family in a negative way. With this approach it will seem that you are pushing your family away in favor of your job. At the end of the day nothing is more important than your family. Do not desert them or orphan them for your job. It is not worth it. Strike a balance, make time for them, and be sure they know how much you love them.

At the end of the day nothing is

more important than your

family. Do not desert them or

orphan them for your job.

It is not worth it.

Chapter 28

Finances

Do not find yourself at the end of residency wondering why you did not partake in any basic preparation to establish a financially stable foundation for yourself and your family.

In full disclosure, I am not a financial adviser and I cannot attest to being the most financially savvy individual throughout medical school and residency. That being said, I would like to offer some very basic words of financial advice that I have learned the hard way.

Collectively as junior physicians we do a terrible job of managing money and few of us receive any dedicated financial education during our medical training. For the large majority of us our formal education is focused on science and medicine, not business or finance. Do not find yourself at the end of residency wondering why you did not partake in any basic preparation to establish a financially stable foundation for yourself and your family.

Putting your financial life in order will take the brain power from this subject and shunt it toward your medical training where the majority of your brain power belongs. With on-line

Putting your financial life in order will take the brain power from this subject and shunt it toward your medical training where the majority of your brain power belongs.

banking, electronic bill payment, and other on-line financial resources, it is pretty easy to put things on auto-pilot. Enroll in automatic bill payment for all of your bills so that the burden is taken off your plate every month and you will not have to give it another thought.

While residents and fellows may not have a lot of money, or make much money during training, if there is any way possible in your budget to start saving or investing I would encourage you to do this as early as possible no matter how small the amount. How to actually invest your money, asset allocation, diversification, risk tolerance, etc., are beyond the scope of this chapter or my expertise. Each of us will have to factor in different variables when beginning a financial plan. There is no one size fits all approach; however, the basic foundation and building blocks of a sound financial plan will be fairly standardized for most folks as they progress through residency

If there is any way possible in your budget to start saving or investing I would encourage you to do this as early as possible no matter how small the amount.

and fellowship training. If you opt to begin investing, find a reputable financial advisor with reasonable fees who adheres to a true fiduciary standard to help you get started.

If you have student loans, consolidate these loans, if applicable, locking them in at the lowest interest rate possible. Make on-time payments each month via automatic electronic withdrawal, as you do for your other bills, and avoid any deferral, forbearance, or grace periods if at all possible. Depending on your particular loan type, interest may continue to accrue during deferral, forbearance, or grace periods without concomitant payments toward the principal sum during that time.

Be smart with your money. Budget, do not overspend, and do not live beyond your means, as you will be living on a resident or fellow salary. Additionally, you will likely have a

Be smart with your money.

Budget, do not overspend, and

do not live beyond your means,

as you will be living on a

resident or fellow salary.

sizeable student loan sum to chisel away at for years to come following completion of your training. Pay off your student debt as quickly as you can and minimize accruing additional debt. Do not dig yourself into a deeper hole during residency or fellowship by purchasing an expensive car or home that you cannot afford before you are actually being paid like a board-certified physician who has completed training and is earning a real salary. Your time will come. Be patient.

I would encourage you to work in concert with your department, training institution, or program director to host an annual personal finance conference or symposium for the residents. A one-day session with a vetted certified financial planner to assist with putting the wheels into motion for building a sound financial base and plan of attack would go a long way for the large majority of medical residents.

If the terms "mutual fund," "index fund," "401-K," "Traditional and Roth IRA," "Thrift Savings Plan," "compound interest," "expense ratios," etc. sound like a foreign language to you, or make you feel a little nervous, then an annual seminar on personal finance associated with your program would no doubt be extremely beneficial. The sooner you can get smart on personal finance, if you are not already savvy on this subject, the better off your financial life will be in the long run.

Take full advantage of and harness the incredible power of compounding interest over your thirty- to forty-year career. Following completion of your training, if you possess a fundamentally sound and firmly entrenched financial foundation, you will be able to tactfully employ your well-deserved earning potential and in turn adeptly grow your investment assets to reach your financial goals. Albert Einstein himself once said, "Compound interest is the eighth wonder of the world. He who understands it, earns it... he who doesn't... pays it." Heed this sage advice from Uncle Al. Last time I checked he is no slouch in the brain power department...

Take full advantage of and harness the incredible power of compounding interest over your thirty- to forty-year career.

Build a secure, long-term financial plan for yourself and your family early on in your professional career and stick to it. You will not regret this. Being disciplined in the financial sector over the course of your training and your career will undoubtedly produce financial independence. The sooner you can get started the better. And as they say, the best time to invest was yesterday.

Part VII

ONGOING EDUCATION

The only constant is change and becoming a lifelong student is the only way to keep up.

Chapter 29

Read one hour per day

Get into the habit of reading some form of medical text one hour per day as often as possible.

One of the most valuable pieces of academic advice I could give a resident in any field of medicine would be to get into the habit of reading some form of medical text one hour per day as often as possible.

There will be a plethora of on-line resources, textbooks, journals, and board preparation materials available to you that are all competing for your attention. The sheer volume of available resources can be overwhelming. It does not have to be. Do not worry yourself with reading through every available resource out there. It is not possible.

Do not worry yourself with reading through every available resource out there. It is not possible.

You will be better served to find one reputable and dominant textbook about your particular specialty that you can read and relate to without falling asleep and drooling after the second sentence. Not all textbooks of medicine and surgery are created equal. What may be easy for one person to read may be a narcoleptic-inducing misadventure for another.

Similarly, you do not need to devour every medical journal that is published in your particular field of practice. You should select a single reputable monthly journal that focuses on your specialty and read it cover to cover every month. This academic

Select a single reputable

monthly journal that focuses on

your specialty and read it cover

to cover every month.

exercise alone will be a huge step in the right direction to keep you academically savvy and up to date with the latest standards of care in your specialty throughout the course of your training and beyond.

In the same vein, when the time comes for in-service examinations or board examinations, focus on one comprehensive board preparation resource and consider attending a seminar on board preparation, written or oral, for your particular specialty. You can use other texts or resources as supplemental information to augment the comprehensive board preparation resource you ultimately select.

If you try to soak up every shred of text that is available you will drive yourself crazy. Focus on a single key textbook and a single professional peer-reviewed journal for your specialty before you take on additional volumes or periodicals.

205

When the time comes for in-service examinations or board examinations, focus on one comprehensive board preparation resource and consider attending a seminar on board preparation, written or oral, for your particular specialty.

If you can regularly engage in one hour of reading daily, or most days of the week, when the time comes for those always looming in-service examinations and board examinations, you will be prepared. The rush to cram when you already have an overwhelmingly busy clinical schedule will not be necessary.

Focus on a single key textbook and a single professional peer-reviewed journal for your specialty before you take on additional volumes or periodicals.

If you are training in a particular medical specialty that requires an oral board examination for your final certification, take the time to practice oral board examination style scenarios with your mentors, colleagues, or attendings throughout your training. If your residency program does not already hold annual or bi-annual "mock oral" examinations for the house officers, you should encourage your program director or chairman to incorporate this into your academic schedule. Do not wait until the end of your residency or fellowship to practice these oral board examination scenarios. The sooner you can begin doing this, no matter how junior you are, it will make a tremendous difference on examination day.

If you are training in a particular medical specialty that requires an oral board examination for your final certification, take the time to practice oral board examination style scenarios with your mentors, colleagues, or attendings throughout your training.

Chapter 30

Research

Try to be involved in some form of academic research, case studies, poster presentations, book chapter contributions, etc. during your training.

While I cannot claim to be a resident who churned out a boat-load of peer-reviewed journal articles, book chapters, or practice-changing research, I was able to scratch out several journal articles and case presentations.

I would encourage all residents to try and be involved in some form of academic research, case studies, poster presentations, book chapter contributions, etc. during your training. It is kind of like exercise during your training, every little bit will help.

Being engaged in research will keep you engaged in academia which you cannot escape in the profession of medicine. It will keep you up to speed with the changes that are constantly occurring around us in medicine at lightning fast speed. If you lose pace with the world of research which ultimately supports new practice guidelines, you will be left behind.

Participating in research as a resident will certainly bolster your fellowship applications should you pursue a fellowship after residency training. It will help you to be competitive in the post-training job market should you pursue an academic faculty position and it will keep your academic prowess sharp.

Even if you are not the first author of a project, fight to become engaged in some form of academic research wherever you are training. Research is painstakingly hard work and publications take time to play out. Stick with it. Apply some of the principles we have discussed previously and it will get done.

If at all possible find a project that you are actually interested in being involved with rather than a topic that you really do not find intriguing. Jumping into a project that you cannot relate to or find any true interest in will be like trying to force a square peg into a round hole. It will be sheer agony. For someone who enjoys bench research, a project involved with trauma surgery may not be very exciting and you will not truly engage with this endeavor.

If at all possible find a project
that you are actually interested
in being involved with rather
than a topic that you really do
not find intriguing.

There are a myriad of research projects ongoing at all times in all training institutions. Seek them out, find something that will engage your mind, and jump right into the fray.

Chapter 31

Professional organizations & societies

All medical trainees should join

at least one major professional

medical society or organization

related to their specialty as a

resident member.

There are a plethora of professional organizations, societies, and conferences throughout the breadth of all medical specialties. I would encourage all medical trainees to join at least one major professional medical society or organization related to their specialty as a resident member. These organizations typically offer resident membership for a nominal cost and it is well worth it.

These organizations have phenomenal opportunities for residents to include leadership positions locally, regionally, and nationally, as well as scholarship opportunities, networking opportunities, and numerous other resources. Some of these other resources include access to newsletters, journals, blogs, and conferences, as well as discounts on conferences, in-service training examination preparation courses, and board certification courses.

I would also encourage and highly recommend all residents in their final year of training to attend the premier annual conference for their particular specialty. This is a fantastic experience in your final year of training as you approach the summit of completing residency training and it is a great experience to share with your fellow residents. Excellent research is presented and cutting-edge technology will be on display. It is motivating to see so many physicians at these conferences who are excited to be pushing the field of medicine forward with leaps and bounds.

If you do not partake in these societal opportunities throughout your training you are truly missing out.

All residents in their final year of training should attend the premier annual conference for their particular specialty.

Part VIII

MENTOR, TEACH, & LEAD

The talented, intelligent, and bright-eyed junior medical trainees that are hitting the clinical wards today will undoubtedly become the leaders, educators, and innovators of our timeless, noble, and altruistic profession tomorrow. Foster their growth in developing a focused posture of confidence, professionalism, and integrity, as well as empathy, humility, and a tireless work ethic as they move forward in their training.

Chapter 32

Mentorship

Having someone in your corner

as an experienced mentor to

draw advice, knowledge, and

assistance from is vital as you

proceed along your own path

and adventure in medicine.

In the profession of medicine, a price truly cannot be placed on the value of a strong mentor-mentee relationship. As we have outlined, medicine is an extremely challenging but rewarding field that is constantly progressing and changing. Having someone in your corner as an experienced mentor to draw advice, knowledge, and assistance from is vital as you proceed along your own path and adventure in medicine. You cannot go it alone. Having a trusted mentor will be invaluable during your formal years of training and beyond.

Having a trusted mentor will be invaluable during your formal years of training and beyond.

Your mentors will have been there, done that, and they will have made the same mistakes you find yourself making. At times they can prevent you from making these potentially shared mistakes and therein lies one of the many values of a good mentor. Sometimes you need to vent, sometimes you need some sense talked into you, and sometimes you need to be recalibrated and berated a little. All of these conversations can happen in a collegial and non-punitive manner with a solid mentor.

A mentor should be someone that you trust, someone you respect and admire, someone with character and integrity, someone who will talk to you straight, and someone who will willingly listen as well as voluntarily provide constructive feedback.

A mentor should be someone that you trust, someone you respect and admire, someone with character and integrity, someone who will shoot you straight, and someone who will willingly listen as well as voluntarily provide constructive feedback.

You do not want your mentor to blow endless rays of sunshine up your rear-end. They should be able to criticize your actions and you need to be receptive to these critiques without putting up a defensive wall or muttering excuse after excuse. Listen to them. They are trying to help you, not belittle you. They can coach you through difficult times, keep you in check if you become arrogant, and keep things objective as an outsider looking in with a fresh set of non-rose-colored spectacles.

While having a mentor is extremely important I also believe it is important to have a mentee no matter how junior you are in your training. A younger generation will sometimes have a better working knowledge of newer data, equipment, and technology that they can educate you about. They will at times provide a fresh and different perspective on how an issue may

While having a mentor is extremely important it is also important to have a mentee, no matter how junior you are in your training.

be approached that maybe you have not thought of before. This will also give you the opportunity to teach, to lead, and to hone these important skills of teaching and leadership.

Take the role of a mentor or mentee seriously and nurture this relationship. You will find that it will be an extremely important, rewarding, and worthwhile relationship during your training and throughout your career to follow.

Take the role of a mentor or mentee seriously and nurture this relationship.

Chapter 33

Teach

Knowledge is power.

We all have the gift of knowledge that we can pass down to those coming up through the ranks below us. This vast bank of knowledge we possess will only grow larger as you progress further through your training and throughout your career. Do not let the knowledge you have gained stagnate and do not keep it to yourself. Spread this wealth of knowledge and teach the folks rising in the ranks below you. Arm them with the same knowledge and lessons learned that you have gained as you have progressed through your training.

There are ample opportunities to teach as a house officer during your medical training no matter how junior you are. Capitalize on these opportunities as often as able. Inpatient rounds are exploited and advertised as the Holy Grail for clinical

We all have the gift of knowledge

that we can pass down to those

coming up through the ranks

below us.

teaching; however, there are other endless opportunities to effectively engage in teaching: in outpatient clinics, in the emergency department seeing patients or consults, in the

There are ample opportunities to

teach as a house officer during

your medical training no matter

how junior you are. Capitalize

on these opportunities as often

as able.

operating room, in academic conferences, or in the wee hours of the night as you dutifully patrol the wards and put out clinical fires along the way. Opportunities for an ad hoc teaching discussion are everywhere. Furthermore, these ad hoc teaching moments in my experience are some of the most valuable teaching moments when they are spur of the moment, spontaneous, or off the cuff. Take advantage of these opportunities whenever you can.

When you find yourself confidently teaching or instructing others, this means you are developing some degree of mastery of what you are teaching or instructing; however, there is always room for improvement. Teaching, whether it is clinical acumen on the wards or technical skills in the operating theater, will make you a better clinician and a better leader. Students will pose questions that you may not have thought of previously, forcing you to delve deeper into a subject for your

Teaching, whether it is clinical acumen on the wards or technical skills in the operating theater, will make you a better clinician and a better leader.

225

own increased understanding. Facts may be challenged by your pupils with a fresh perspective. Your students may bring valuable new insight to the fundamental understanding of a problem or they may foster a novel approach to a process that will improve upon it from the long-accepted norm.

The enduring value, positive impact, inspiring influence, and rewards of teaching are infinite. A resident who does not actively pursue regular teaching and instruction of those coming through the training pipeline below them is truly missing a vital opportunity for their own personal development and is forgetting a key central pillar of medical training.

Chapter 34

Lead

We will let you make mistakes

but we won't let you fail.

When you become a house officer, you automatically become a leader whether you realize it or not, or whether you want to or not. Embrace it. When you are an intern you are a leader to the medical students, when you are a junior resident you are a leader to the interns, when you are a chief resident or fellow you are a leader to the residents, and when you become an attending you are a leader to all tiers of medical training.

In addition to your clinical prowess or technical abilities in the profession of medicine, leadership is a skill you should strive to be a student of and continuously hone as you progress in your career.

When you are an intern you are a

leader to the medical students,

when you are a junior resident

you are a leader to the interns,

when you are a chief resident or

fellow you are a leader to the

residents, and when you become

an attending you are a leader to

all tiers of medical training.

Medical trainees at all levels thirst for leadership, they thirst for knowledge, and they are looking for you to provide that leadership whether you want to or not. Embrace this role and use it to actively develop your own personal leadership skills. It will pay dividends for the rest of your career. Your leadership efforts will no doubt shape and mold the next generation of medical leaders and innovators.

Push those under you to improve but also be patient with them, listen to them, and encourage them no matter how bad

Leadership is a skill you should

strive to be a student of and

continuously hone as you

progress in your career.

of a day you are having yourself. Can you put aside your own problems momentarily to listen to a colleague or help one of your junior trainees work through a difficult problem they are having? A leader will do this.

As you progress through your medical training learn to pluck positive leadership traits from those attendings, mentors, and senior residents that you respect and admire. Soak up everything you can from them. You will easily recognize these positive leadership traits when you witness them. More so, and even easier to identify, are the negative leadership traits that you will not want to emulate.

Be stern, decisive, and firm when it is warranted but also be fair and objective when dealing with peers or trainees who need their priorities or perspective rearranged as a result of poor performance or disciplinary problems. You should be stern when it is required to institute corrective actions of an individual or individuals but do not be an outright jerk. There is a distinct difference.

As you progress through your medical training learn to pluck positive leadership traits from those attendings, mentors, and senior residents that you respect and admire.

Maintain an even keel and avoid going high and right at the first sign of trouble. Those who can keep a cool head when a situation begins to deteriorate toward chaos and can keep a team of healthcare providers working as one cohesive and effective unit are good leaders.

If you take care of your medical students and junior residents, they will go to extreme lengths to take care of you. If you treat them poorly they will do the same to you in return. When you are a solid and respectable leader, those coming up in the ranks below you will become all out mercenaries on a war against pathology and your team will succeed no matter what challenges are thrown your way.

Those who can keep a cool head

when a situation begins to

deteriorate toward chaos and can

keep a team of healthcare

providers working as one cohesive

and effective unit are good leaders.

One of the most inspiring quotes I heard during my training which I think reflects true leadership is, "We will let you make mistakes but we will not let you fail." As a leader you cannot micromanage those who work with you and those whom you are training. One of the best teachers in life is to be able to make mistakes and to actively learn from these mistakes.

Allow your team members to put themselves out there as you yourself need to put yourself out there to succeed. It is no different. Sure, they are going to make mistakes. A mistake will demonstrate a valuable point or lesson learned to the individual who committed the mistake, as well as to the other trainees, and it will be incorporated into the active learning process. It is your job as a leader to recognize when one of your peers or trainees commits a mistake that requires your active intervention. Then you may assist them in working through a tough situation and circumvent overt failure. Allow them to make mistakes but do not let them fail.

Strive to leave your training program better off than the way you found it. Everyone has something to give back to a department or training program that will improve the quality of the end product. This can be a number of things such as completing valuable research for the department, gaining a research grant for your program, collaboration with other training programs, fostering societal affiliations through leadership positions, performing process improvement projects, and recruiting solid house officers to the program.

Be a solid leader that your junior residents, peers, attendings, department, and patients can look up to and lean on when the going gets tough. Inspire those around you with infectious optimism, perpetual energy, and intrepid drive.

Be a solid leader that your junior residents, peers, attendings, department, and patients can look up to and lean on when the going gets tough.

Afterword

If you continue to employ the same professional characteristics, positive attitude, steadfast morals, and tireless work ethic we have discussed in these chapters, you will continue to be wildly successful well beyond residency or fellowship.

During the process of writing this book, and as I have transitioned from residency into junior attending life, I have pondered the next steps along my career path. I have asked myself the question, "What will make me a successful physician and professional moving forward?"

Ultimately, I realized the answer to this rhetorical question was really pretty simple. What will make me, or any other physician, who is transitioning from residency or fellowship into their attending years successful are the same traits that made you successful in residency and I hope to have effectively highlighted these attributes in this book. If you continue to employ the same professional characteristics, positive attitude, steadfast morals, and tireless work ethic we have discussed in these chapters, you will continue to be wildly successful well beyond residency or fellowship.

The world is your oyster as long as you provide some form of righteous substrate for it to work with. I would argue that the primary substrate to begin synthesis are the fundamental "three As": availability, affability, and ability. Tack on a few side chains of perseverance, endurance, mental strength, fortitude, integrity, and empathy to the "three As" and the rest will take care of itself. This will be the scaffold for you to begin building upon layer after layer of successes and ultimately create an invaluable pearl that will be illustrative of your career as a successful and self-fulfilled physician, mentor, teacher, and leader.

You will never truly know what situations, epic experiences, or grand adventures life will deal you along the way. Never let your guard down and be ready for whatever wild cards end up in your hand for better or for worse. Some of these wild cards will be your ace in the hole and some will flat out suck. Be ready for both.

Never let your guard down and be ready for whatever wild cards end up in your hand for better or for worse.

Live in the moment, take it one step at a time, be the best you can be with each small step along the way, and you will succeed. Amazing opportunities will find their way to you. With the tools we have discussed in this book you will translate these opportunities into epic adventures and successes that you can continue to build upon and polish throughout your career as a respected physician and well-rounded professional.

Live in the moment, take it one

step at a time, be the best you

can be with each small step

along the way, and you

will succeed.

It is out there waiting for you. I wish you fair winds and following seas. Now take the helm and get to it!